ACSM's
Health/Fitness Facility Standards and Guidelines

American College of Sports Medicine

Editors

Stephen J. Tharrett, MS, ACSM Program Director®
Consultant, Dallas, TX

Kyle J. McInnis, ScD, FACSM
University of Massachusetts, Boston, MA

James A. Peterson, PhD, FACSM
Healthy Learning, Monterey, CA

Human Kinetics

Library of Congress Cataloging-in-Publication Data

American College of Sports Medicine.
  ACSM's health/fitness facility standards and guidelines / ACSM : Stephen J.
Tharrett, editor, Kyle J. McInnis, editor, James A. Peterson, editor. -- 3rd ed.
      p. ; cm.
  Includes bibliographical references and index.
  ISBN-13: 978-0-7360-5153-8 (hard cover)
  ISBN-10: 0-7360-5153-8 (hard cover)
  1. Physical fitness centers--Standards--United States.   2. American College of
Sports Medicine.
  [DNLM: 1. Physical Education and Training--standards--United States--Guideline.
2. Physical Fitness--United States--Guideline.   3. Health Facilities,
Proprietary--standards--United States--Guideline.   QT 255 A5135 2006]   I. Title:
Health/fitness facility standards and guidelines.   II. Tharrett, Stephen J., 1953-
III. McInnis, Kyle J.   IV. Peterson, James A., 1943-   V. Title.
  GV429.A45 2006
  613.7'1--dc22   2005033377

ISBN-10: 0-7360-5153-8

ISBN-13: 978-0-7360-5153-8

The Web addresses cited in this text were current as of June 28, 2006, unless otherwise noted.

Acquisitions Editor: Michael S. Bahrke, PhD; **Developmental Editor:** Amanda S. Ewing; **Assistant Editor:** Carmel Sielicki; **Copyeditor:** Jan Feeney; **Proofreader:** Sarah Wiseman; **Indexer:** Betty Frizzéll; **Permission Manager:** Dalene Reeder; **Graphic Designer:** Robert Reuther; **Graphic Artist:** Kathleen Boudreau-Fuoss; **Cover Designer:** Keith Blomberg; **Art Manager:** Kelly Hendren; **Illustrators:** Gretchen Walters; art in supplements 12 and 16 by Denise Lowry; art in appendixes C and D by Andrew Tietz; **Printer:** Sheridan Books

ACSM Publication Committee Chair: Jeffrey L. Roitman, EdD, FACSM
ACSM Group Publisher: D. Mark Robertson
ACSM Editorial Assistant: David J. Wanaselja

Human Kinetics books are available at special discounts for bulk purchase. For details, contact the Special Sales Manager at Human Kinetics.

Printed in the United States of America   10   9   8   7   6   5   4   3   2   1

Human Kinetics
Web site: www.HumanKinetics.com

United States: Human Kinetics, P.O. Box 5076, Champaign, IL 61825-5076
800-747-4457
e-mail: humank@hkusa.com

Canada: Human Kinetics
475 Devonshire Road Unit 100, Windsor, ON N8Y 2L5
800-465-7301 (in Canada only)
e-mail: orders@hkcanada.com

Europe: Human Kinetics
107 Bradford Road, Stanningley, Leeds LS28 6AT, United Kingdom
+44 (0) 113 255 5665
e-mail: hk@hkeurope.com

Australia: Human Kinetics
57A Price Avenue, Lower Mitcham, South Australia 5062
08 8277 1555
e-mail: liaw@hkaustralia.com

New Zealand: Human Kinetics
Division of Sports Distributors NZ Ltd., P.O. Box 300 226 Albany, North Shore City, Auckland
0064 9 448 1207
e-mail: info@humankinetics.co.nz

CONTENTS

EDITORS AND EDITORIAL BOARD

PREFACE

The benefits of engaging in a physically active lifestyle are both numerous and well documented. To achieve these benefits in a safe and efficient manner, however, people should adhere to a few well-defined training principles and guidelines while exercising. Furthermore, it can be extremely useful for an individual to have access to resources (e.g., fitness equipment and well-designed exercise programs) that can help ensure a positive exercise experience. Having access to and contact with professionally trained personnel who can facilitate the proper use of those tools via direct instruction or supervision can be helpful in this regard.

Not surprisingly, millions of people have chosen to join health/fitness facilities (such as YMCAs, Jewish Community Centers, health/fitness clubs, and corporate fitness centers) that can provide them with the tools and exercise environment that they perceive that they need to be physically active. All factors considered, the better managed these facilities are, the more likely they will be to provide their users with exercise experiences that are safe, time-efficient, and effective.

The focus of the efforts surrounding the development of the three editions of *ACSM's Health/Fitness Facility Standards and Guidelines* has been to establish a blueprint that specifies what health/fitness facilities must do to maintain the standard of care that they offer their members and users, and what health/fitness facilities should provide in order to enhance the exercise experience that members and users can achieve by taking advantage of the activities and programs offered by a particular facility. Before the publication of three editions of this landmark text, no such blueprint existed.

To fulfill its role as the most respected sports medicine and exercise science professional organization in the world, the American College of Sports Medicine (ACSM) assumed the responsibility of leadership with regard to providing operators of health/fitness facilities with a clearly defined set of recommended practices to promote safe exer-

cise participation. In 1990, in response to guidance given by the ACSM president at that time, Dr. Lyle Micheli, ACSM initiated the process of assembling a team of experts in the academic, medical, and health/fitness fields to develop and write a manual on standards and guidelines for delivering quality physical activity programs and services to consumers. In 1992, the product of the collective efforts of that team was published as a text on standards and guidelines for designing and operating a health/fitness facility. The comprehensive nature of that work was reflected in its 353 separate standards plus an additional 397 guidelines.

Approximately five years after the first edition of *ACSM's Health/Fitness Facility Standards and Guidelines* was published, a number of steps were undertaken to evaluate the need for and the format of a second edition of the book. The primary action in this regard was the appointment of an ad hoc committee of leaders from the medical, exercise science, and health/fitness facility communities to discuss and study the matter. The committee subsequently issued a consensus report that concluded that a second edition of the book was needed to resolve various industry, professional, and consumer-oriented concerns. The committee felt that a second edition of the book would enable the information in the text to be updated, while allowing essential features of the publication to be reorganized into what was designed to be a more balanced format. Compared with the first edition, the revised work would place greater emphasis on taking into account the views and input of industry trade organizations and of a wide variety of fitness associations. In this regard, the primary focus was to develop a document that would be more reflective of a true consensus of the health/fitness industry.

In response to the findings of the ad hoc committee, ACSM appointed a committee to develop a second edition of *ACSM's Health/Fitness Facility Standards and Guidelines,* which was published in 1997. In an attempt to gain broader support in the health/fitness industry, the second edition featured a number of major changes from the first edition.

First and foremost, the myriad of standards and guidelines presented in the first edition were consolidated into six standards and approximately 500 guidelines. Responding to a charge given by the ACSM committee that reviewed the first edition, the editorial committee for the second edition reduced the original list of 353 standards that must apply to all health/fitness facilities to six standards. In contrast to the original open-ended tabulation of standards, the six standards identified in the second edition offered a condensed, more realistic focus concerning the standard of care that must be demonstrated by all health/fitness facilities toward their users.

In contrast to the substantial reduction in the number of standards that were detailed in the second edition, the total number of guidelines increased by more than 20%. Designed to serve as possible tools for health/fitness facility owners and managerial staff to improve their operations, these guidelines set forth design considerations and operating procedures that, if employed, would enhance the quality of service that a facility provides to its users. The guidelines were not intended to be standards of practice or to give rise to duties of care. Finally, the second edition featured augmented appendixes.

In 2004, approximately eight years after the publication of the second edition of *ACSM's Health/Fitness Facility Standards and Guidelines*, a committee of industry-wide representatives and exercise science professionals selected by ACSM recommended that not only would a third edition of this benchmark text be appropriate, but it was also clearly needed. Since research had shown that many health/fitness facilities were not complying with the recommendations set forth in the previous editions of the book, it would be helpful if additional clarifications and application-related information were included to accompany each recommendation. Another factor was the need for relevant recommendations concerning the development of the technological advances offered by such devices as automated external defibrillators (AEDs). This third edition

of this text is the result of that decision and a by-product of the efforts that followed.

In contrast to the first two editions of this book, the third edition is organized into chapters that feature a review and discussion of specific focal points. Each chapter addresses both the standards and guidelines that pertain to a particular issue.

Chapter 1 provides an overview of the updated standards and guidelines for health/fitness facilities. Chapter 2 addresses pre-activity screening, and chapter 3 examines orientation, education, and supervision. Chapter 4 offers a greatly expanded section on risk management and emergency procedures. Chapter 5 covers professional staff and independent contractors. Chapters 6, 7, and 8 catalog issues involving design and construction, equipment, and operational practices, respectively, in health/fitness facilities. Chapter 9 provides an overview of factors concerning signage in a health/fitness facility. Finally, the number of supplemental materials and forms included in the appendixes has been substantially increased over the two previous editions of the book.

In every possible instance, an effort has been made to include text in the third edition of this book that can help health/fitness facilities be prepared to adhere to the required standards and to adopt the recommended guidelines. To the extent that these materials can enhance the ability of health/fitness facilities to provide quality service and program offerings in an appropriate environment, the potential importance of this book cannot be overestimated.

Finally, as with the two previous editions of this text, this book is intended to provide standards and guidelines for pre-activity screening, orientation, education, and supervision, risk management and emergency procedures, professional staff and independent contractors, facility design and construction, facility equipment, operational practices, and signage. It is not intended to present general exercise standards and guidelines. The fundamental principles of sound exercise programming and prescription are relatively well documented and readily available elsewhere.

ACKNOWLEDGMENTS

The American College of Sports Medicine and the editors of this third edition of *ACSM's Health/Fitness Facility Standards and Guidelines* would like to extend their thanks to the members of the editorial board who committed their time and expertise to the writing of this book. Additional thanks are extended to the editors of the two previous editions of this book—Carl Foster, PhD, and Neil Sol, PhD, on the first edition and James A. Peterson, PhD, and Stephen J. Tharrett, MS, on the second edition—for their foresight in helping establish the legacy of this book.

The editors would also like to extend a special thanks to the ACSM Board of Trustees for their contribution to and involvement in the establishment of this book and its predecessors. For more than 50 years, ACSM has played a leading role in the growth in the level of professionalism exhibited by the industry.

Finally, special thanks are extended to the organizations that reviewed the draft manuscript for this book and provided the editors with feedback on its content.

NOTICE AND DISCLAIMER

The American College of Sports Medicine's (ACSM) purpose for developing the previous and current editions of this book is to enhance the safety and effectiveness of physical activity conducted in health/fitness facilities, with the goal of increasing global participation rates in physical activity. To this end, the book will address pre-activity screening practices, orientation, education, and supervision issues, risk management and emergency-procedure practices, staffing issues, design and facility issues, equipment issues, operational practices, and signage issues that have an impact on the safety and effectiveness of physical activity as conducted by the general population in health/fitness facilities.

ACSM and its senior co-editors and editorial board, in setting forth standards and guidelines in this book, have done so based on the following definitions for standards and guidelines.

- **Standards.** These are base performance criteria or minimum requirements that ACSM believes each health/fitness facility must meet to satisfy a facility's obligations to provide a relatively safe environment in which every physical activity or program is conducted in an appropriate manner. These standards are not intended to give rise to duty of care or to establish a standard of care; rather, they are performance criteria derived from a consensus of ACSM leaders. The standards are not intended to be restrictive nor to supercede national, regional, or local laws and regulations and are qualitative in nature. Finally, as base performance criteria, these standards are steps designed to promote quality and to accommodate reasonable variations, based on local conditions and circumstances.

- **Guidelines.** These are recommendations that ACSM believes health and fitness operators should consider using to improve the quality of the service they provide to users. Such guidelines are not standards, nor are they applicable in every situation or circumstance; rather, they are illustrative tools that

ACSM believes should be considered by health and fitness operators.

ACSM and its senior co-editors and editorial board have designed this book as a resource for those who operate all manner of health/fitness facilities, whether they be fully staffed facilities or unstaffed and unsupervised facilities, such as some hotel fitness centers, worksite centers, and commercial facilities. Some of the standards and guidelines detailed in this book, in particular those that apply to issues of staffing and supervision or the execution of a practice requiring staffing, may not be applicable to those facilities whose operational model does not include facility staffing.

Despite the development and publication of this book, the responsibility for the development and delivery of services and procedures remains with the facility that is providing services. Individual circumstances may necessitate deviation from these standards and guidelines, such as a facility that is not staffed. Facility personnel must exercise professionally derived decisions as to what is appropriate for individuals or groups under particular circumstances. These standards and guidelines represent ACSM's opinion regarding best practices. Responsibility for service provision is a matter of personal and professional experience.

Any activity, including those undertaken within a health/fitness facility, carries with it some risk of harm, no matter how prudently and carefully services may be provided. Health/fitness facilities are not insurers against all risks of untoward events; rather, their mission should be directed at providing facilities and services in accordance with applicable standards. The standard of care that is owed by facilities is ever changing and emerging. As a consequence, facilities must stay abreast of relevant professional developments in this regard.

By reason of authorship and publication of this document, neither the editors, the authors, nor the publisher are, or shall be deemed to be, engaged in the practice of medicine or any allied health field, the practice of delivering fitness training services, or the practice of law or risk management. Rather, facilities and professionals must engage the services of appropriately trained and/or licensed individuals to obtain those services.

The words *safe* and *safety* are frequently used throughout this publication. Readers should recognize that the use of these terms is relative and that no activity is completely safe.

Blueprint for Excellence

The primary purpose of this book is to provide a blueprint that can help facilitate the need of health/fitness facilities to provide a relatively safe environment for those who engage in the activities and programs offered by the facility and can ensure that these offerings are conducted in an appropriate manner. Accordingly, this chapter lists 21 standards and 36 guidelines that apply to health/fitness facilities.

Collectively, these standards and guidelines are further addressed in chapters 2 to 9, grouped and dealt with by topic (pre-activity screening; orientation, education, and supervision; risk management and emergency policies; professional staff and independent contractors; facility design and construction; equipment; operating practices; signage). Each chapter presents both an overview of the standards and guidelines attendant to a particular topic and a discussion of the rationale underlying each standard and guideline.

Tables 1.1 and 1.2 provide a list of the standards and guidelines, respectively, that have been identified as appropriate for health/fitness facilities. The chapter in which each standard and guideline is covered is noted in parentheses following each specific listing.

TABLE 1.1 Standards for Health/Fitness Facilities

1. All facilities offering exercise equipment or services must offer a general pre-activity cardiovascular risk screening, e.g., Physical Activity Readiness Questionnaire (PAR-Q) and/or a specific pre-activity screening tool, e.g., health risk appraisal (HRA), health history questionnaire (HHQ), to all new members and prospective users (chapter 2).

2. All specific pre-activity screening tools (e.g., HRA, HHQ) must be interpreted by qualified staff and the results of the screening must be documented (chapter 2).

3. If a facility becomes aware that a member or user has a known cardiovascular, metabolic, or pulmonary disease, or two or more major cardiovascular risk factors, or any other major self-disclosed medical concern, as a result of a pre-activity screening, that person must be advised to consult with a qualified healthcare provider before beginning a physical activity program (chapter 2).

4. All facilities with qualified staff must offer each new member a general orientation to the facility, including identification of resources available for personal assistance with developing a suitable physical activity program and the proper use of any exercise equipment to be used in that program (chapter 3).

5. Facilities must have in place a written system for sharing information with users and employees or independent contractors regarding the handling of potentially hazardous materials, including the handling of bodily fluids by the facility staff in accordance with the Occupational Safety and Health Administration (OSHA) (chapter 4).

6. Facilities must have written emergency response systems policies and procedures,

which must be reviewed and rehearsed regularly, as well as documented. These policies must enable staff to handle basic first-aid situations and emergency cardiac events (chapter 4).

7. Facilities must have as part of their written emergency response system a public access defibrillation (PAD) program (chapter 4).

8. The fitness and healthcare professionals who have supervisory responsibility for the physical activity programs (supervise and oversee members, users, staff, and independent contractors) of the facility must have an appropriate level of professional education, work experience, and/or certification (chapter 5).

9. The fitness and healthcare professionals who serve in counseling, instructional, and physical activity supervision roles for the facility must have an appropriate level of professional education, work experience, and/or certification (chapter 5).

10. Fitness and healthcare professionals engaged in pre-activity screening, instructing, monitoring, or supervising of physical activity programs for facility members or users must have current automated external defibrillation and cardiopulmonary resuscitation (AED and CPR) certification from an organization qualified to provide such certification (chapter 5).

11. Facilities, to the extent required by law, must adhere to the building design standards that relate to the designing, building, expanding, or renovating of space as presented by the Americans with Disabilities Act (ADA) (chapter 6).

12. Facilities must be in compliance with all federal, state, and local building codes (chapter 6).

13. The aquatic and pool facilities must provide the proper safety equipment and signage according to state and local codes and regulations (chapter 7).

14. Facilities must have a system in operation that monitors the entry to and usage of the facility by all individuals, including members and users (chapter 8).

15. Facilities that offer a sauna, steam room, or whirlpool must ensure that these areas are maintained at the proper temperature and that the appropriate warning systems are in place to notify members and users of any unacceptable risks and changes in temperature (chapter 8).

16. Facilities that offer members and users access to a pool or whirlpool must ensure that the pool water chemistry is maintained in accordance with state and local codes (chapter 8).

17. A facility that offers youth services or programs must provide appropriate supervision (chapter 8).

18. Facilities must post the appropriate caution, danger, and warning signage in conspicuous locations where existing conditions and situations warrant such signage (chapter 9).

19. Facilities must post the appropriate emergency and safety signage pertaining to fire and related emergency situations, as required by federal, state, and local codes (chapter 9).

20. Facilities must post all required ADA and OSHA signage (chapter 9).

21. All cautionary, danger, and warning signage must have the required signal icon, signal word, signal color, and layout, as specified by the American National Standards Institute (ANSI) and reflected in the American Society of Testing and Materials (ASTM) standards for fitness equipment and fitness facility safety signage and labels (chapter 9).

TABLE 1.2 Guidelines for Health/ Fitness Facilities

1. All screening procedures should be rapid, simple, and easy to perform; the process should encourage acceptance of the opportunity to participate in the pre-activity screening (chapter 2).

2. Prospective members and users who fail to complete the pre-activity screening procedures on request should be permitted to sign a waiver or release that allows them to participate in the program offerings at the facility. In those instances where such members and/or users refuse to sign a release or waiver, they should be excluded from participation to the extent permitted by law (chapter 2).

3. All members and users who are identified as having cardiovascular or medical risk factors that merit medical consultation should be provided with appropriate information concerning the importance of obtaining such consultation from a qualified healthcare provider before beginning an exercise program (chapter 2).

4. All members and users who have been identified (either through pre-activity screening or

by self-disclosure) as having cardiovascular, metabolic, or pulmonary disease or symptoms or any other potentially serious medical concern (e.g., orthopedic problems) and who subsequently fail to get a consultation should be permitted to sign a waiver or release that allows them to participate in the facility's program offerings. In those situations where such members and users refuse to sign a waiver or release, they should be excluded from participation to the extent permitted by law (chapter 2).

5. Facilities should offer each member or user of a health/fitness facility either a general physical activity orientation or information that can facilitate that person's participation in the physical activity programs of the facility (chapter 3).

6. Facilities should provide new and existing members with the opportunity to receive personal instruction and guidance with their physical activity programs (chapter 3).

7. Facilities should provide members with ongoing monitoring of their physical activity programs, including the opportunity to receive guidance on adjusting their physical activity program (chapter 3).

8. Staffed facilities should provide professional fitness staff to supervise the fitness floor during peak usage periods (chapter 3).

9. Depending on their targeted audience, facilities should consider providing an array of physical activity options to accommodate the physical, emotional, and personal preferences of each user of the facility (chapter 3).

10. Facilities should validate that their employees and independent contractors who are involved in providing health and fitness assessments, fitness, and lifestyle counseling and instruction, personal training, massage, health and fitness advice or related professional service have the requisite education, certification, and experience to safely and effectively perform the responsibilities of their jobs (chapter 4).

11. Facilities should perform criminal background checks on employees and independent contractors who have responsibilities that involve working with youth or whose responsibilities involve personal contact with members and users or other employees in an unsupervised environment (chapter 4).

12. Facilities should use waivers of liability and/or assumption-of-risk documents with all facility members and users (chapter 4).

13. Facilities should have an incident report system for written documentation of all incidents that occur within the facility or within the facility's scope of responsibility. Such reports should be completed in a timely fashion and maintained on file according to the statute of limitations for the government district in which they do business (chapter 4).

14. A facility that delivers or prescribes physical activity programs primarily or exclusively to members and users who are considered at an elevated risk for incurring a health-related problem because of their participation in physical activity (e.g., users over the age of 50 or with coronary risk factors, diabetes, or clinical obesity) should have a medical liaison or medical advisory committee that assists in reviewing physical activity screening and programming protocols as well as emergency response protocols (chapter 5).

15. Facilities should provide the appropriate level of supervision and monitoring for each of the physical activity areas in the facility (chapter 5).

16. A facility should extend to each employee on staff the opportunity to receive training and certification in first aid and use of CPR and AED (chapter 5).

17. Facilities should allocate sufficient space for physical activity zones so that defined circulation routes are adjacent to, rather than through, the physical activity areas (chapter 6).

18. Facilities should provide open-access circulation, which avoids blind corners, unnecessary doors, pointless partitions, and other hazards that would present a safety risk to members and users (chapter 6).

19. Facilities should separate physical activity spaces from operational, storage, and maintenance spaces (chapter 6).

20. Facilities should design both physical activity spaces and nonactivity spaces so as to provide sufficient space to accommodate the expected user demand placed on each space within the facility (chapter 6).

21. Facilities should provide all physical activity spaces with sufficient air circulation and fresh make-up air (i.e., outside air), which will allow the facility to maintain air quality, room temperature, and humidity at safe and comfortable levels during times of physical activity (chapter 6).

22. Facilities should properly illuminate all facility spaces in order to allow members and users to

safely navigate the various facility spaces and perform their physical activity regimens. Minimum safe illumination levels vary according to activity and should be carefully researched. The emerging need for energy conservation requires lighting solutions that take advantage of the available daylighting sources, automatic control devices, and the latest technologies in lamp and fixture design (chapter 6).

23. Facilities should be designed to maintain background noise levels below 70 decibels and never above 90 decibels. Sound transmission through defining perimeter partitions of a noise-generating activity area should be limited to a level that does not adversely affect the functionality of neighboring spaces (chapter 6).

24. Floor surfaces in physical activity areas should provide the proper level of absorption and slip resistance to minimize the risk of users' incurring impact or fall-related injuries (chapter 6).

25. Facilities should have wall surfaces in activity spaces that are nonabrasive, flush, and free of protrusions that could cause impact injuries. Activity spaces that involve airborne projectiles, such as volleyballs and basketballs, should have a perimeter ball-containment barrier to protect users in adjacent areas and walkways (chapter 6).

26. When physical activity spaces have depth or distance parameters that can affect an individual's safety, then the facility should provide the appropriate markings to ensure that users are aware of these depth-and-distance parameters (chapter 6).

27. Facilities should provide a sufficient quantity and quality of equipment so that the facility is able to fulfill its mission, purpose, and intended function for its targeted members and users (chapter 7).

28. Facilities should have a preventive maintenance program for their fitness equipment, including documentation showing when the scheduled work was performed (chapter 7).

29. All physical activity areas should have a clock, a chart of target heart rates, and a chart depicting ratings of perceived exertion to enable members and users to monitor their level of physical exertion (chapter 7).

30. Facilities that are staffed during all operating hours should have a manager on duty (MOD) or supervisor on duty (SOD) schedule that specifies which professional staff person has supervisory responsibility overseeing all operating activities during the hours that the facility is open (chapter 8).

31. Facilities should provide the proper level of qualified staffing in nonactivity areas to assist in serving the members and users and providing support to emergency response situations that might arise (chapter 8).

32. Facilities that are unstaffed during some or all operating hours, and therefore have periods in which no supervision is offered, should provide the appropriate signage to communicate to members and users that the facility is unsupervised, the inherent risks in using the facility, and what steps the members and users should take in the event of a witnessed emergency situation (chapter 8).

33. Facilities should have a written system for cleaning and disinfecting the various areas in the facility (chapter 8).

34. Facilities should attempt to provide every activity area in the facility with the appropriate safety and warning signage (chapter 9).

35. Facilities should provide message boards, bulletin boards, or similar signage for the communication and dissemination of relevant information on the facility or of particular interest to the facility's members (chapter 9).

36. Signage should have the proper appearance, readability, and placement in order to clearly display the desired message in a fashion that can easily be understood by the intended audience (chapter 9).

Table 1.3 offers a list of key terms and their definitions as they apply in this text.

TABLE 1.3 Key Terms and Their Definitions

Guidelines are recommendations that ACSM believes health and fitness operators should consider using to improve the quality of the service they provide to users. Such guidelines are not standards, nor are they applicable in every situation or circumstance. Rather, they are illustrative tools that ACSM believes should be considered by health and fitness operators.

Health/fitness facility member is an individual who pays either monthly dues or annual dues for the privilege of engaging in the activities, programs, and services of the facility. Members maintain the privileges of membership for as long as they pay dues, with a predetermined minimum time period, normally one month. In essence, a member has entered into a contractual agreement with the health and fitness facility to access its activities, programs, and services in return for paying membership dues. In many cases, members have access to multiple facilities operated by the same facility-ownership group.

Health/fitness facility user is an individual who accesses a facility on one and possibly more than one occasion without purchasing a membership to the facility. In most cases, the user is an individual who has received a complimentary guest pass or has paid for a guest pass to gain one day's or one week's access to the facility. A user has no contractual arrangement with the facility other than having access for a given time period, normally ranging from one day to one week, and in rare instances for a set number of visits associated with enrollment in a special program.

Standards are base performance criteria or minimum requirements that ACSM believes each health and fitness facility must meet to satisfy a facility's obligations to provide a relatively safe environment in which every physical activity or program is conducted in an appropriate manner. Furthermore, these standards are not intended to give rise to duty of care or to establish a standard of care; rather, they are performance criteria derived from a consensus of ACSM leaders. The standards are qualitative in nature and are not intended to be restrictive or to supercede national, regional, or local laws and regulations. Finally, as base performance criteria, they are steps designed to promote quality and to accommodate reasonable variations, based on local conditions and circumstances.

With regard to addressing the issue of to which organizations or groups the standards should apply, it is important to note that ACSM has not attempted to define precisely what types of physical activities and programs collectively constitute a facility. It is the position of ACSM that any business or entity that provides an opportunity for individuals to engage in activities that may reasonably be expected to involve placing stress on one or more of the various physiological systems (cardiovascular, muscular, thermoregulatory) of the body must adhere to the 21 standards detailed in this text.

CHAPTER 2

Pre-Activity Screening

The promotion of physical activity is an important focus of the national public health agenda in America. In that regard, the time and resources that are devoted to encourage people to be physically active are supported by an ever-accumulating and impressive body of scientific literature that documents the innumerable health benefits of a physically active lifestyle and the potential detrimental effects of sedentary living. As a result of the public health message that individuals should regularly engage in moderate to vigorous physical activity, an increased level of interest and participation in fitness facilities has occurred, including the involvement of adults with diverse health and medical conditions and relatively low levels of cardiorespiratory fitness.

Other factors, such as an aging population, a twin epidemic of obesity and type 2 diabetes, and efforts to promote physical activity to the "beginner fitness" population, have heightened the need for careful safety policies and procedures that are put into practice at all health/fitness facilities. The primary intent of such policies and procedures is to minimize cardiovascular and/or medical risk for all members and users, including those at greatest potential for cardiovascular risk during exercise due to their age, presence of existing cardiovascular disease, symptoms or risk factors, and any other medical concern that might otherwise be exacerbated during exercise participation.

Although most individuals are at very low risk for an exercise-related cardiovascular event, such as sudden cardiac death or acute myocardial infarction, accumulating scientific evidence suggests the risk of adverse cardiac events is considerably higher during or immediately after exercise, especially in habitually sedentary individuals who engage in unaccustomed vigorous physical activity. The risk of a cardiovascular event is highest in persons with occult or known heart disease. However, these individuals are difficult to identify, since many individuals who experience exercise-related cardiovascular emergencies have no previous warning signs.

An important challenge facing health/fitness facilities is to provide the proper environment for stimulating interest and motivation toward exercise participation while simultaneously minimizing the potential risk of an adverse medical event occurring during or soon after exercise. A vitally important procedure involved in optimizing safe exercise participation is to identify those individuals who may be at an increased risk for such events. The primary step in achieving that objective is to routinely administer a pre-activity health risk assessment on all new members and prospective users. Accordingly, individuals deemed to be at an increased cardiovascular and/or medical risk can be properly evaluated by qualified healthcare providers and steered toward activities that are consistent with their health needs and receive specific recommendations about exercising safely and their potential activity limitations.

Pre-activity screening is the method by which a health/fitness facility can properly identify those members and users who pose an increased risk of experiencing exercise-related cardiovascular incidents. This procedure is necessary for providing would-be exercisers with appropriate guidelines and recommendations for safe and effective exercise participation. This chapter presents standards and guidelines pertaining to the use of pre-activity screening protocols in health/fitness facilities. Table 2.1 lists the three required standards for pre-activity screening; table 2.2 details the guidelines for pre-activity screening.

Standards for Pre-Activity Screening

TABLE 2.1 Standards for Pre-Activity Screening

1. All facilities offering exercise equipment or services must offer a general pre-activity cardiovascular risk screening, e.g., Physical Activity Readiness Questionnaire (PAR-Q) and/or a specific pre-activity screening tool, e.g., health risk appraisal (HRA), health history questionnaire (HHQ), to all new members and prospective users.

2. All specific pre-activity screening tools (e.g., HRA, HHQ) must be interpreted by qualified staff and the results of the screening must be documented.

3. If a facility becomes aware that a member or user has a known cardiovascular, metabolic, or pulmonary disease, or two or more major cardiovascular risk factors, or any other major self-disclosed medical concern, as a result of a pre-activity screening, that person must be advised to consult with a qualified healthcare provider before beginning a physical activity program.

Pre-activity screening standard 1. All facilities offering exercise equipment or services must offer a general pre-activity cardiovascular risk screening, e.g., Physical Activity Readiness Questionnaire (PAR-Q) and/or a specific pre-activity screening tool, e.g., health risk appraisal (HRA), health history questionnaire (HHQ), to all new members and prospective users.

The primary purpose of pre-activity screening is to identify those known to be at risk for an adverse event during exercise and those who should undergo an appropriate medical evaluation before starting an exercise program. This objective involves identifying persons with known cardiovascular disease, symptoms of cardiovascular disease, diabetes or other risk factors for disease development, or other

major health conditions that may affect safe exercise participation. Screening also identifies persons with known cardiovascular disease or other special medical needs who should ideally participate, at least initially, in a medically supervised program.

Pre-activity screening tools can be either general (meaning they provide a generic and simple means of identifying primary cardiovascular risk factors) or specific (meaning they provide a more in-depth approach to identifying preexisting health conditions). The most commonly used general pre-activity screening tool is the Physical Activity Readiness Questionnaire (PAR-Q), which was developed by the Canadian Heart Association. The PAR-Q is a simple one-page questionnaire that asks questions that allow the user or a facilitator to easily identify major health conditions, signs or symptoms suggestive of coronary heart disease, risk factors for cardiovascular disease, medications, or other major medical conditions that may elevate the participant's risk of medical complications during exercise. (Refer to form 1 in appendix B for a sample PAR-Q.)

A commonly used form of a more specific pre-activity screening tool is a health risk appraisal (HRA) questionnaire, of which there are many varieties. HRAs range from simple one-page questionnaires to more complex questionnaires that focus on identifying the health risks associated with an individual's fitness, health, and lifestyle choices. Another commonly used type of a specific pre-activity screening tool is a medical history questionnaire (HHQ), of which there are also numerous versions. Due to the greater detail in items that are normally included in HRAs and HHQs, the usefulness of these tools is greatly facilitated when the instruments are used with the assistance of fitness or healthcare professionals who have sufficient education and knowledge to interpret the findings and make appropriate recommendations. (Refer to form 2 in appendix B for a sample HHQ.)

Pre-activity screenings (either general or specific) can either be self-administered by the user or conducted by a fitness or healthcare professional. A self-administered, general pre-activity screening is most appropriate for health/fitness facilities that are unstaffed during all or part of their operating hours, such as hotel fitness centers, apartment fitness centers, and even some commercial health and fitness facilities. A self-administered pre-activity screening protocol can range from the posting of a PAR-Q with accompanying signage at the entry to a health and fitness facility to a PAR-Q form being distributed to each facility user at his or her first visit to the facility and having them complete it. Pre-activity screenings (either general or specific) that are facilitated by a fitness or healthcare professional are most suitable for health and fitness facilities that are staffed and focused on providing additional physical activity guidance to users. Furthermore, members and users must be offered the pre-activity screening prior to their participation. The pre-activity screening may be repeated at appropriate intervals.

Pre-activity screening standard 2. All specific pre-activity screening tools (e.g., HRA, HHQ) must be interpreted by qualified staff, and the results of the screening must be documented.

It is essential that suitable information be collected on whether participation in physical activity presents a heightened cardiovascular and/or medical risk for a prospective member or user of a health/fitness facility. It is also critical that such information be appropriately interpreted and the results be used to make appropriate decisions about what constitutes safe activity levels for that particular individual.

Pre-activity screening standard 3. If a facility becomes aware that a member or user has a known cardiovascular, metabolic, or pulmonary disease, or two or more major cardiovascular risk factors, or any other major self-disclosed medical concern, as a result of a pre-activity screening, that person must be advised to consult with a qualified healthcare provider before beginning a physical activity program.

Once a member or user has completed a facility-administered pre-activity screening protocol, the facility must have a system in place that recommends evaluation from a qualified healthcare provider, if indicated. The American College of Sports Medicine (ACSM) has developed a practical approach to risk stratification that can be used to classify individuals as low, moderate, or high risk. This stratification can be subsequently used to provide recommendations for receiving further evaluation from a qualified healthcare provider. Risk-classification schemes (as adapted from the ACSM) that can be used for guiding decisions about making recommendations for medical evaluation are presented in appendix G.

For self-administered pre-activity screening protocols that are used by health/fitness facilities, the form can advise the respondent to seek medical advice. For facilities that choose to use the PAR-Q, the interpretation can be performed simply by recommending a specific course of action (e.g., seek further evaluation from a qualified healthcare provider or professional).

One approach to providing clearance or approval is to make use of a medical clearance or physician's recommendation form that addresses the advisability of and conditions for an exercise program in which that particular user might engage. These are forms that users can take to a personal physician to obtain the physician's approval to engage in physical activity. In accordance with the Health Insurance Portability and Accountability Act of 1996 (HIPAA), facilities may not be able to release a user's health information directly to a physician or other healthcare professional without first receiving the permission of the user. As a result, if a user needs to receive medical clearance before participating in a particular activity program, it is prudent and helpful for the facility to provide the appropriate forms to the user to take to a physician. Sample forms, consistent with HIPPA requirements and that serve this purpose, are presented in forms 4 and 5 in appendix B.

Guidelines for Pre-Activity Screening

TABLE 2.2 Guidelines for Pre-Activity Screening

1. All screening procedures should be rapid, simple, and easy to perform; the process should encourage acceptance of the opportunity to participate in the pre-activity screening.

2. Prospective members and/or users who fail to complete the pre-activity screening procedures on request should be permitted to sign a waiver or release that allows them to participate in the program offerings of the facility. In those instances where such members and/or users refuse to sign a release or waiver, they should be excluded from participation to the extent permitted by law.

3. All members and users who are identified as having cardiovascular or medical risk factors that merit medical consultation should be provided with appropriate information concerning the importance of obtaining such consultation from a qualified healthcare provider before beginning an exercise program.

4. All members or users who have been identified (either through pre-activity screening or by self-disclosure) as having cardiovascular, metabolic, or pulmonary disease or symptoms or any other potentially serious medical concern (e.g., orthopedic problems) and who subsequently fail to get consultation should be permitted to sign a waiver or release that allows them to participate in the facility's program offerings. In those situations where such members or users refuse to sign a waiver or release, they should be excluded from participation to the extent permitted by law.

Pre-activity screening guideline 1. All screening procedures should be rapid, simple, and easy to perform; the process should encourage acceptance of the opportunity to participate in the pre-activity screening.

All prospective members and users should be informed about the value of participating in pre-activity screening. Appropriate steps should be taken to facilitate such acceptance.

Pre-activity screening guideline 2. Prospective members and users who fail to complete the pre-activity screening procedures on request should be permitted to sign a waiver or release that allows them to participate in the program offerings at the facility. In those instances where such members and/or users refuse to sign a release or waiver, they should be excluded from participation to the extent permitted by law.

On occasion, some members or users may not want to participate in the facility's pre-activity screening protocol. While research indicates that completing a pre-activity screening protocol may be beneficial in identifying medical conditions that might expose a member or user to a heightened risk of experiencing a cardiovascular incident during or soon after physical activity, members have the freedom to determine if participating in pre-activity screening is best for them. To reduce the facility's liability, it is advisable that such member or user be asked to sign a waiver or release, where permissible by law, that clearly indicates that the person has been offered a pre-activity screening and that (a) this member or user has been informed of the risks of participation; (b) this member or user

has chosen not to follow the guidance provided; (c) this person assumes personal responsibility for his or her actions; and (d) this individual releases the facility from any claims or suits arising from his or her participation. If the member or user signs the waiver or release, that person should be afforded the opportunity to participate in a physical activity program at the facility. If the member or user chooses not to sign the waiver or release, the facility has the option of denying that person the privilege to participate or access to the facility to the extent permitted by law. (Refer to form 6 in appendix B for a sample waiver.)

Pre-activity screening guideline 3. All members or users who are identified as having cardiovascular or medical risk factors that merit medical consultation should be provided with appropriate information concerning the importance of obtaining such consultation from a qualified healthcare provider before beginning an exercise program.

The need by individuals with certain identifiable risk factors to receive medical consultation from a qualified healthcare provider before they engage in a moderate to vigorous exercise program should be thoroughly explained to those prospective members or users. In a clear, easy-to-understand manner, the explanation should address why it is in the best interests of such individuals to obtain appropriate medical consultation. The necessity for medical consultation is particularly critical for those individuals with predetermined medical conditions (such as coronary heart disease, diabetes, arthritis, and obesity) that involve special needs. In fact, those health and fitness facilities that primarily (or exclusively) serve such populations should be particularly aware of the value of pre-activity screening involving oversight by qualified personnel.

Pre-activity screening guideline 4. All members or users who have been identified (either through pre-activity screening or by self-disclosure) as having cardiovascular, metabolic, or pulmonary disease or symptoms or any other potentially serious medical concern (e.g., orthopedic problems) and who subsequently fail to get consultation should be permitted to sign a waiver or release that allows them to participate in the facility's program offerings. In those situations where such members or users refuse to sign a waiver or release, they should be excluded from participation to the extent permitted by law.

When used properly, a pre-activity screening protocol will help determine when a person who may be at increased cardiovascular or medical risk during moderate to vigorous exercise participation could benefit from receiving consultation from a qualified healthcare provider. It is always in the member's or user's and facility's best interests to strongly encourage those individuals to obtain the proper medical consultation. It should be noted that there may be instances in which a member or user may not have any known or apparent medical risk factors or symptoms. The facility may still consider it in the best interest of that individual to receive medical consultation before participating in the facility's program offerings.

On occasion, members or users may refuse to obtain recommended medical clearance. When that situation occurs, where legally permissible, the facility should secure a waiver and release that clearly indicates that (a) the users have been informed of the risks of participation and that they have been instructed to obtain medical clearance, (b) they have chosen not to follow the guidance provided, (c) they assume personal responsibility for their actions, and (d) they release the facility from any claims or suits arising from their participation.

If the member or user signs the waiver or release, that person should be afforded the opportunity to participate in physical activity program offerings at the facility. In the event the member or user chooses not to sign the waiver or release, the facility may chose to deny that individual the privilege of participating in the facility's program offerings or access to the facility to the extent permitted by law.

Orientation, Education, and Supervision

The orientation, education, and supervision of members and users in a health/fitness facility are some of the most important obligations a facility has to those individuals it serves. Orientation refers to the process of providing each facility member or user with the proper information and guidance to initiate and engage in a program of safe and effective physical activity. Education involves the practice of facilities providing relevant, up-to-date information to their members and users so that these individuals can make informed decisions about their physical activity and lifestyle practices. Supervision is the process of monitoring the physical activity practices of members and users so that the physical activity environment promotes safe participation.

Several market studies have been conducted that indicate that although more than 80% of Americans are aware of the benefits of being physically active, only 20% actually engage in physical activity on a regular basis. This discrepancy between what Americans know about the benefits of physical activity and their actual behavior patterns serves to reinforce the need for health/fitness facilities to engage in practices that help orient, educate, and supervise users.

This chapter presents standards and guidelines on the orientation, education, and supervision of members and users. Table 3.1 lists the one required standard on orientation, education, and supervision; table 3.2 details the five recommended guidelines for orientation, education, and supervision.

Standards for Orientation, Education, and Supervision

TABLE 3.1 Standards for Orientation, Education, and Supervision

1. All facilities with qualified staff must offer each new member a general orientation to the facility, including identification of resources available for personal assistance with developing a suitable physical activity program and the proper use of any exercise equipment to be used in that program.

Orientation, education, and supervision standard 1. All facilities with qualified staff must offer each new member a general orientation to the facility, including identification of resources available for personal assistance with developing a suitable physical activity program and the proper use of any exercise equipment to be used in that program.

Once a member has completed a pre-activity screening process, the health/fitness facility must then provide the member with a general orientation to the facility. A general orientation can take many forms, including any of the following:

• **Group orientation classes.** In facilities that have a low staff-to-user ratio or who have a high volume of member traffic, providing a schedule of orientation classes that users can select from can be a viable option. These orientation classes should be offered at various times to allow members and users the opportunity to attend. Among the topics that these orientation classes could cover are basic instructions concerning how members and users should use the various pieces of physical activity equipment that are available in the facility. In addition, these classes could review what resources are available within the facility that can help members and users develop a suitable physical activity program (e.g., personal training services, special fitness classes, fitness media library, online personal training experts). Finally, these classes can even provide an introduction to a general physical activity regimen that members and users can follow.

• **Personal orientation sessions.** The ideal situation for any member is to receive a personal orientation from a qualified fitness professional. This offering allows the individuals to receive advice and guidance firsthand from a qualified fitness professional. The personal orientation should include general guidelines on physical activity, a personalized exercise regimen that is based on the user's pre-activity screening results and predetermined goals, and a hands-on walk-through of that individual's physical activity regimen.

Guidelines for Orientation, Education, and Supervision

Table 3.2 Guidelines for Orientation, Education, and Supervision

1. Facilities should offer each member or user of a health/fitness facility either a general physical activity orientation or information that can help facilitate that person's participation in the physical activity programs of the facility.

2. Facilities should provide new and existing members with the opportunity to receive personal instruction and guidance with their physical activity programs.

3. Facilities should provide members with ongoing monitoring of their physical activity programs, including the opportunity to receive guidance on adjusting their physical activity program.

4. Staffed facilities should provide professional fitness staff to supervise the fitness floor during peak usage periods.

5. Depending on their targeted audiences, facilities should consider providing an array of physical activity options to accommodate the physical, emotional, and personal preferences of each user of the facility.

Orientation, education, and supervision guideline 1. Facilities should offer each member or user of a health/fitness facility either a general physical activity orientation or information that can help facilitate that person's participation in the physical activity programs of the facility.

Health/fitness facilities should offer information to their members and users that can help enhance the level of safety, efficiency, and participation in the facility's physical activity offerings. Among the approaches that could be considered in this regard are the following:

• **Provide orientation signage and literature.** In facilities that are either unsupervised or not supervised at all times, the use of signage and literature that outline the proper steps for engaging in safe physical activity can be very helpful. For example, this approach could involve having facilities provide some basic guidelines (e.g., dos and don'ts) for engaging in physical activity, as well as a basic physical activity regimen that a facility's users could follow. Another example would be to ensure that instructional decals are posted on the exercise equipment that detail how to use the devices safely. The manufacturers of most exercise equipment include such decals as standard issue.

• **Make orientation information available on the facility's Web site.** Health/fitness facilities can provide basic orientation information on selected areas or files on its Web site, which its members and users can access. The information can be offered in several formats, including texts, images, and streaming video. Depending on the available technology, members and users should also have the option of downloading the information.

• **Conduct orientation classes.** A facility can offer scheduled classes that provide information to enhance the exercise experience of its members and users.

Orientation, education, and supervision guideline 2. Facilities should provide new and existing members with the opportunity to receive personal instruction and guidance with their physical activity programs.

While not always possible, personal instruction and targeted guidance that a qualified fitness professional can provide members will normally result in better safety and productivity than would otherwise be achieved in a given physical activity program. On the other hand, industry-based research shows that only between 5 and 10% of members and users of a facility receive personalized exercise instruction (referred to in the industry as *personal training*) on a regular basis. This low level of individualized attention is due at least in part to the costs involved in having a fitness professional fulfill that particular role. One way that facilities can help create a greater level of personalized instruction is by offering options that include the following:

- **Complimentary follow-up orientations.** Facilities can offer new members and current members the opportunity for complimentary 30-minute personal sessions at predetermined intervals (e.g., their 90-day membership anniversary and again at one-year intervals).

- **Fee-based private sessions.** Facilities can offer members the opportunity to purchase the services of a qualified fitness professional who could provide them with ongoing instruction and guidance.

- **Web-based personalized private instruction.** Facilities can align themselves with one of the Web-based personal training systems that allow members to interact with a qualified fitness professional via e-mail.

Orientation, education, and supervision guideline 3. Facilities should provide members with ongoing monitoring of their physical activity programs, including the opportunity to receive guidance on adjusting their physical activity programs.

Once members and users begin their physical activity programs, their challenge becomes twofold: (a) adhering to the program for a sustained period of time and (b) achieving their intended program-based health/fitness objectives. Facilities can assist members with both of these challenges by providing a system of monitoring a person's physical activity. One of the more common physical activity moni-

toring systems employed by the health and fitness industry involves the use of exercise cards. With exercise cards, members can document their physical activity practices, the results of which can later be reviewed by the facility's professional fitness staff. In the event the fitness professional sees a need for an adjustment in a member's exercise regimen or notes any unusual circumstances that merit further attention, the member can be contacted and appropriate recommendations can be made.

Another monitoring practice within the health and fitness industry that has gained in popularity in recent years is the use of computer software–based monitoring systems. These systems allow members to record their physical activity efforts in electronic format. The results are then reviewed, as needed, by the professional fitness staff, who can then follow up with the individual, either electronically or in person. In the event that a facility does not have sufficient staff to implement either of the aforementioned monitoring programs, they could provide their members with either semiannual or annual pre-activity screenings, the results of which could be used to help monitor members on a regular basis.

Orientation, education, and supervision guideline 4. Staffed facilities should provide professional fitness staff to supervise the fitness floor during peak usage periods.

During the highest usage periods within a facility, it is recommended that at least one qualified fitness professional be made available on the fitness floor to assist members and users with any questions they may have, to provide guidance when needed, and to respond to any potential emergency situations that might arise. While no ratio currently exists for the number of members and users to professional fitness staff, it is advisable that there be at least one freestanding fitness professional (i.e., an individual who is not engaged in providing users with personalized instruction) for every 100 facility users.

Orientation, education, and supervision guideline 5. Depending on their targeted audiences, facilities should consider providing an array of physical activity options that accommodate the physical, emotional, and personal preferences of each user of the facility.

It is not easy to start and stay with a program of physical activity, as evidenced by studies showing that more than 50% of new exercisers drop out within 90 days of beginning an exercise program. Research on physical activity attitudes and behavior, as well as market research conducted by the health and fitness industry, clearly shows that one approach does not fit all when it comes to physical activity programs. Specific to their targeted membership, facilities have a vested interest in getting and keeping their members involved in the activities offered by a particular facility. Accordingly, facilities need to provide a variety of programs to meet the needs of the marketplace, including:

- **Social-based programs.** Many new and existing members prefer to participate in socially based physical activity programs. (Note: This type of programming is in the top five preferences for women.) As a result, facilities should consider offering physical activity programs (such as group exercise classes, tennis leagues, group lessons, group personal training) that feature and foster a component of social interaction in exercise.

- **Competitive-based programs.** Many first-time members and existing members seek a challenge and a competitive outlet within their physical activity pursuits. (Note: This factor is among the top five reasons for men to be motivated to exercise.) As a result, facilities should consider including competitive-based activities, such as sports competitions and events (e.g., basketball, squash), fitness challenges (e.g., bench press contests, running events), and personal goal-oriented programs (e.g., weight loss, etc.) in their facility.

- **Health and wellness programs.** As stated by members and users, as well as nonusers, among the top reasons for participating is the need for participants to improve their level of health and well-being. As a result, a facility's offerings should include programs targeted toward health and well-being, such as back education classes, arthritis exercise classes, and nutrition classes.

- **Mind–body programs.** Over the past few years, there has been an escalating demand for program offerings that feature a mind–body approach to activity or an approach that focuses on achieving a balance between physical activity and relaxation. According to market research, women are particularly interested in these types of activities, as are older adults. Among the examples of these types of physical activity programs are Pilates, tai chi, and yoga.

- **Weight loss and weight management programs.** Numerous studies indicate that losing weight is one of the primary reasons many people join health/fitness facilities. This factor, combined with the alarming rise in obesity among Americans, is more than sufficient reason that facilities should consider incorporating such popular programs as weight loss, weight management, and nutrition education in their program offerings.

Facilities should also consider serving as a resource for their members with regard to the body of knowledge attendant to fitness, health, and wellness. As such, facilities can help keep their members informed about the current facts pertaining to fitness, health, and wellness. Unfortunately, health/fitness facility members, as well as all individuals in our society, are constantly bombarded in the media with misinformation about fitness, health, and wellness. As a result, an objective source of information is needed that can help these individuals sort out the information on these topics as it directly applies to their personal needs. Facilities can provide this information in several ways, including:

- **Communication media.** Facilities can provide their users with important information on fitness and health education through the use of various media. For example, newsletters that have a section devoted to the dissemination of fitness and health information are one viable means of communicating essential information. Web sites that have an education page or link to a fitness and health Web site are another way to help members get the information that they need. Finally, a health/fitness facility can use a bulletin board or other similar display on which articles on fitness and health can be posted.

- **Classes, clinics, and workshops.** Facilities should consider offering classes, clinics, and workshops on specific fitness and health-related topics to their members and users. For example, a facility could offer a monthly health education seminar series featuring health and fitness professionals from the community who speak on topics such as cardiovascular health and women's health issues. Another example would be for a facility to have its own professional staff offer a series of workshops on timely and important fitness- and health-related topics, such as weight management, back-care education, healthy eating, stress management, and exercise and arthritis.

Risk Management and Emergency Policies

Risk management refers to the practices and systems that businesses put in place to reduce or limit their exposure to liability and financial loss. In the fitness and health club industry, risk management refers to the practices, procedures, and systems by which the club reduces its risk of having an employee, member, or user experience an event that could result in harm (injury or death) to the individual (employee, member, or user) and perhaps later to the business entity itself. Risk management covers practices that range from those that are preventive in nature (such as pre-activity screening and properly caring for equipment) to those practices that are considered a reaction or a recovery-and-response system to untoward events (such as emergency response systems).

This chapter presents standards and guidelines for the risk management and emergency procedures that health/fitness facilities need to consider in order to provide a safe physical activity environment for its employees, members, and users. Some of the standards and guidelines that might otherwise be considered risk management practices, such as pre-activity screening and other operational practices, are addressed in other chapters of this book. Table 4.1 lists three required standards for risk management and emergency policies; whereas table 4.2 details the four recommended guidelines for risk management and emergency policies.

Standards for Risk Management and Emergency Policies

TABLE 4.1 Risk Management and Emergency Policy Standards

1. Facilities must have in place a written system for sharing information with users and employees or independent contractors regarding the handling of potentially hazardous materials, including the handling of bodily fluids by the facility staff in accordance with the standards of the Occupational Safety and Health Administration (OSHA).

2. Facilities must have written emergency response system policies and procedures, which must be reviewed and rehearsed regularly, as well as documented. These policies must enable staff to handle basic first-aid situations and emergency cardiac events.

3. Facilities must have as part of their written emergency response system a public access defibrillation (PAD) program.

Risk management and emergency policies standard 1. Facilities must have in place a written system for sharing information with users and employees or independent contractors regarding the handling of potentially hazardous materials, including the handling of bodily fluids by the facility staff in accordance with the standards of the Occupational Safety and Health Administration (OSHA).

The health and fitness industry is one that can expose members and users, employees, and independent contractors to materials that OSHA considers dangerous. Employees and independent contractors, such as custodial staff, lifeguards, locker room and fitness staff, and others, may be exposed to chemicals and materials that are potentially hazardous, such as cleaning agents, paints, and lubricants. Those individuals who are in enclosed areas where air circulation is limited can be exposed to particle matter, such as debris resulting from sanding, drilling, or similar activity. To comply with OSHA guidelines and reduce the risk to users and staff, facilities need to consider the following actions:

- Make sure that the material safety data sheet (MSDS) for every chemical and agent used in the facility is posted in a location for all workers to see.

- Provide an MSDS binder for each staff person to review and have each person sign appropriately to signify that he or she has reviewed the information and understands the issues.

- Store all chemicals and agents in proper locations. Ensure that these materials are stored off the floor and in an area that is off limits to users. These areas should also have locks to prevent accidental or inappropriate entry.

- Provide regular training to workers in the handling of these items.

- Post the appropriate signage to warn users that they may be exposed to these hazardous agents.

The health and fitness facility industry is one that may expose its users and staff to various bodily fluids. Almost every human interaction associated with this industry has the potential to result in contact with bodily fluids. As such, the possibility exists that disease-producing organisms may be present in those fluids. Consequently, exposure carries a risk of infection. The OSHA standard on bloodborne pathogens addresses how such fluids must be handled to minimize risks of infection. Many facility operators fail to realize that even the handling of towels presents an increased risk of exposure to bodily fluids such as blood or perspiration. Some key steps that every facility can take to minimize risk in this area include the following:

- Provide appropriate training for staff. Make sure that all staff are taught how to handle bodily fluids. OSHA provides training materials, as do other organizations.

- Provide literature to staff on the handling of bodily fluids.

- Make sure that the staff members who are handling towels, cleaning or picking up papers, and cleaning exercise equipment wear surgical-style gloves. Staff that have to handle bar soap or razors also need to be provided with latex gloves or similar type of gloves.

- Make sure that the facility has a system for disposing of items containing bodily fluids. If the facility has razors, then a biowaste container for disposing of them must be provided. If facility personnel are washing towels, bleach must be used since it will kill most pathogens carried in bodily fluids.

If blood is visible, it must be cleaned off immediately with bleach or similar agent while wearing barrier protection apparel (e.g., impermeable gloves). All cleaning materials and all fluids must be disposed of in biowaste containers. Untrained staff should not be permitted to handle these materials or fluids. Full details on the OSHA Hazard Communication Standard are included in appendix A, supplement 5.

Risk management and emergency policies standard 2. Facilities must have written emergency response system policies and procedures, which must be reviewed and rehearsed regularly, as well as documented. These policies must enable staff to handle basic first-aid situations and emergency cardiac events.

Having an emergency response system is critical to providing a safe environment for members and users and staff as well as being a sound practice in risk management. For health/fitness facilities, emergency response systems must be developed in order to provide the highest reasonable level of safety for members and users. Emergency policies, procedures, and practices for health/fitness facilities, as presented and discussed in this chapter, are derived from recommendations published jointly in 1998 and 2002 by ACSM and AHA. (Refer to appendixes G and H.)

Many of these recommendations are identified and discussed in this chapter in the context of standards for health/fitness facilities in 2005 and beyond. However, it is acknowledged that the types of facilities vary markedly, from facilities that are essentially hotel amenities to medically supervised clinic exercise centers. Such facilities often serve different aims and clientele, may or may not have organized program offerings, and may or may not have qualified staff. Thus, beyond the standards offered in this chapter, facilities needing assistance in matters of preparing emergency policies, procedures, and practices relevant to their setting will find the contents of the 1998 and 2002 ACSM/AHA publications to be helpful resources. Among the more crucial elements attendant to incorporating emergency response systems in a facility are the following:

- Facilities should use local healthcare or medical personnel to help them develop their emergency response program. Most local emergency medical services will assist a facility in developing its response program. Facilities can also pay for the services of a physician, registered nurse, or certified emergency medical technician to guide the development of their emergency response program.

- The emergency response system must address the major emergency situations that might occur. Among those situations that might occur are those medical emergencies that are reasonably foreseeable with the onset of moderate or more intense exercise, such as hypoglycemia, sudden cardiac arrest, heart attack, stroke, heat illness, and those injuries that are orthopedic in nature. The response system must also address other foreseeable emergencies not necessarily associated with physical activity, such as fires or chemical accidents.

- The emergency response system must provide explicit steps or instructions on how each emergency situation will be handled and the roles that should be played by first, second, and third responders to an emergency. In addition, the emergency response system needs to provide locations for all emergency equipment (e.g., telephone for 911 or other

contact information for EMS, the location for all emergency exits, and the most favorable access ways for the EMS personnel, as well as the steps necessary for contacting the local EMS).

- The emergency response system must be fully documented (i.e., staff training, emergency instructions) and kept in an area that can be easily accessed by the club staff. In addition, the emergency response system needs to be reviewed with each staff person on a regular basis.

- The emergency response system must be physically rehearsed at least four times per year, with notations maintained in a log book that indicate when the rehearsals were performed and who participated.

- The emergency response system must address the availability of first-aid kits and other medical equipment within the facility.

- The emergency response system should identify a local coordinator (e.g., a staff person who is responsible for a facility's overall level of emergency readiness).

Risk management and emergency policies standard 3. Facilities must have as part of their written emergency response system a public access defibrillation (PAD) program.

A PAD program uses automated external defibrillators (AEDs), which are sophisticated computerized machines that are simple to operate and enable a layperson with minimal training to administer this potentially lifesaving intervention. AEDs allow a layperson responding to an emergency to use the AED device, which can detect certain life-threatening cardiac arrhythmias and then administer an electrical shock that can restore the normal sinus rhythm. AED's are the third step in the American Heart Association's (AHA's) renowned Chain of Survival concept, after alerting EMS and administering CPR. Helpful suggestions concerning the important features of PAD programs and resources to assist facilities with integrating the PAD program in their emergency response protocols may be found at the AHA Web site at www.americanheart.org.

Research reviewed by the AHA shows that the delivery speed of defibrillation, as offered by an AED, is the major determinant of success in resuscitative attempts for ventricular fibrillation (VF) cardiac arrest (the most common type of cardiac arrest). Survival rates after VF decrease 7% to

10% with every minute of delay in defibrillation. A survival rate as high as 90% has been reported when defibrillation is administered within the first minute of cardiac arrest, but survival decreases to 50% at five minutes, 30% at seven minutes, 10% at nine to eleven minutes, and 2% to 5% after twelve minutes.

Communities that have incorporated AED use in their emergency practices have shown significant improvements in survival rates for individuals who have experienced cardiac events. In the state of Washington, the survival rate increased from 7% to 26%; in Iowa, the survival rate increased from 3% to 19%. Some public programs have reported survival rates as high as 49% with prompt administration of an AED. The American Heart Association is a strong proponent of having AEDs as accessible to the public as possible. The use and application of AEDs in a public setting are detailed in the American Heart Association's 2000 *Guidelines for Emergency Cardiac Care*. A revised version of the guidelines is scheduled to be released in 2005.

At the present time, use of AEDs in the health and fitness industry has remained somewhat controversial. In 2003, for example, the International Health, Racquet and Sportclub Association (IHRSA) released a position statement on AEDs that indicated that while the Association thought that facilities should consider the installation of an AED, it did not think that AEDs should be mandated for health/fitness facilities. The AHA and ACSM released a joint position statement in 2002 that recommended the implementation of AEDs in health/fitness facilities (appendix H). At this point, five states (Arkansas, Illinois, Rhode Island, New York, and Louisiana) have passed legislation that require health/fitness facilities to have AEDs. In the future, more states are expected to pass legislation requiring health/fitness facilities to provide access to AEDs. In reality, most of the premier health/fitness facility operators in the United States have already made AEDs an integral part of their emergency response systems. Among the basic steps health/fitness facilities might consider in implementing a PAD program for their facility are the following:

- Every site with an AED should strive to get the response time from collapse caused by cardiac arrest to defibrillation to four minutes or less.

- AEDs in a facility should be located within a 1.5-minute walk of a potential collapse site.

- The Food and Drug Administration (FDA) requires that a physician prescribe an AED before it can be purchased. The AHA strongly recommends that a physician, licensed to practice medicine in the community in which the facility is located, should provide the oversight of the facility's emergency system and AEDs. In most cases, the company from which an AED is purchased will assist the facility with identifying a physician to provide these services. Physician oversight refers to the following:

  - Prescribing the AED

  - Reviewing and signing off on the emergency plan

  - Witnessing at least one rehearsal of the emergency plan and indicating so in writing

  - Providing standing orders for use of the AED

  - Reviewing documentation from any instances when the emergency plan is initiated and the AED is used

- A club's emergency plan and AED plan should be coordinated with the local emergency medical services (EMS) provider. (Note: Most of the product providers offer this.) Coordinating with the local EMS provider refers to the following:

  - Informing your local EMS provider that your club has an AED or AEDs

  - Informing your local EMS provider of the location of each AED at the facility

  - Working with the local EMS provider to provide ongoing training of the facility's staff in the use of the AED

  - Working with the local EMS provider to provide monitoring and review of AED events

- A skills review and practice sessions with the AED should be held every six months, as recommended by the AHA's Emergency Cardiac Care Committee and a number of international experts. AED practice drills every three months are recommended for health/fitness facilities.

- The AED should be monitored and maintained according to the manufacturer's specifications on a daily, weekly, and monthly basis, and all information in that regard should be carefully documented and maintained as part of the facility's emergency response system records. Currently, available AEDs provide this function through an automated process.

- All incidences involving the administration of an AED must be recorded and then reported to the physician who is providing oversight as soon as possible, but no longer than one day. (The HIPAA Act does not allow medically sensitive information to be released to anyone other than the medical director.)

- Each club should have an AED program coordinator who is responsible for all aspects of the emergency plan and the use of the AED, as outlined in the standards of care detailed in this book.

- All staff likely to be put in a situation where they may have to administer an AED should be appropriately trained and certified in a course that incorporates the administration of the AED from an accredited training organization. Currently, the AHA and the American Red Cross (ARC) provide AED basic life support training and certification that involve a minimum of four hours of direct-contact training. AHA training and certification last two years, while the corresponding American Red Cross (ARC) program lasts for one year. Records of training and retraining should be maintained in staff personnel records or as part of the documentation of the facility's emergency response system.

- A facility must have at least one employee on duty at all times who is currently trained and certified in BCLS and administration of an AED.

- There are 4 special situations regarding the use and application of an AED that a facility's emergency response team must be familiar with and that are reviewed during initial training: water, children, transdermal medication, and implanted pacemaker or ICD.

- It should be noted that the AHA will release its new guidelines for emergency cardiac care in 2005, and it is expected that some of these guidelines will change from those highlighted in the 2000 edition of the AHA publication referenced in this text.

An effective and rapid PAD system actually depends on bystanders' participating in rapid recognition of potential sudden cardiac arrest and deployment of an AED for possible use. For this reason, health/fitness facilities are encouraged to work with their medical directors and EMS support systems to carefully define prudent and appropriate ways to include all facility members and users in the emergency response system. This process may include consideration of how members and users might be involved directly or indirectly in accessing and deploying the AED and at what point during the emergency protocol that step may be required (e.g., sudden collapse of an individual and no staff member is immediately present). Written instructions might be provided to every member or user concerning the approved PAD program in the facility, what the bystander or user response should be in an emergency, and where the AED is located. Likewise, orientation of new facility members might include a simple printed information card indicating the location of pertinent emergency response postings in the facility; the locations of the emergency telephone and AED; which staff members may need to be employed to handle an emergency, and where their offices are located, should EMS activation be needed.

The orientation for new users could also include visits to locations in the facility to point out areas that are listed on the emergency response information card they have been given. While it is recognized that developing an appropriate way to involve all users in a PAD program will need to be developed carefully and thoughtfully, this process may help to reduce the time between cardiac arrest and defibrillation, when the cause of collapse is ventricular fibrillation, especially in medium to large facilities during those times when member, user, and staff presence is minimal.

Guidelines for Risk Management and Emergency Policies

TABLE 4.2 Guidelines for Risk Management and Emergency Policies

1. Facilities should validate that their employees and independent contractors who are involved in providing health and fitness assessments, fitness and lifestyle counseling and instruction, personal training, massage, health and fitness advice, or related professional service have the requisite education, certification, and experience to safely and effectively perform the responsibilities of their job.

2. Facilities should perform criminal background checks on employees and independent contractors who have responsibilities

that involve working with youth or whose responsibilities involve personal contact with members and users or other employees in an unsupervised environment.

3. Facilities should use waivers of liability and/or assumption of risk documents with all facility members and users.

4. Facilities should have an incident report system for written documentation of all incidents that occur within the facility or within the facility's scope of responsibility. Such reports should be completed in a timely fashion and maintained on file, according to the statue of limitations for the government district in which they do business.

Risk management and emergency policies guideline 1. Facilities should validate that their employees and independent contractors who are involved in providing health and fitness assessments, fitness and lifestyle counseling and instruction, personal training, massage, health and fitness advice, or related professional services have the requisite education, certification, and experience to safely and effectively perform the responsibilities of their job.

The health and fitness industry has numerous positions that require specific personal licensing, registration, or certification for an employee to be considered qualified to serve in the capacity for which that individual has been hired. Facilities can limit their risk by insuring (both at the time of employment or contract signing and during the course of work) that each employee's and independent contractor's credentials are valid and current. If a position that requires special education, training, registration, or licensure is found to be lacking in the individual holding that position, a facility is exposing itself to considerable risk. Examples of positions where credentials need to be checked at the time of employment or contract signing and on an ongoing basis thereafter include fitness instructor, fitness director, personal trainer, group exercise instructor, massage therapist, esthetician, and dietitian. Chapter 5 provides details on some of the specific educational, certification, licensing, and experience requirements for several of the professional roles that exist within a facility and the expectations for documenting current qualifications of employees.

Risk management and emergency policies guideline 2. Facilities should perform criminal

background checks on employees and independent contractors who have responsibilities that involve working with youth or whose responsibilities involve personal contact with members or users or other employees in an unsupervised environment.

In many states, this guideline is often required by law. The employees and independent contractors in the health and fitness industry are actively involved in providing personalized experiences that can expose themselves and the facility to considerable risk. For example, personal trainers, massage therapists, fitness instructors, swim instructors, lifeguards, and others often work closely with users in a one-on-one environment where a risk of an adverse situation exists. Some employees such as child care workers, swim instructors, summer camp instructors, and tennis instructors are in positions in which they work closely with young adults and children in a relationship that often involves some authority or control. These situations and those jobs in which personal contact might occur are positions for which a facility should consider background checks to ensure that these employees have no prior record of unusual behavior that may expose other employees or members and users to harm. A simple background check, performed by an outside law enforcement agency, can determine if a potential employee or independent contractor has a criminal record that might present risk to other employees or members and users. Background checks can take many forms. As it applies to this guideline, a background check is a process that examines whether an employee or independent contractor has a history of criminal behavior indicating inappropriate behavior with adults or children.

Risk management and emergency policies guideline 3. Facilities should use waivers of liability and/or assumption of risk documents with all facility members and users.

An expressed assumption of risk is a legal document that the members and users sign, which indicates they are aware of the risks associated with their participation in the various physical activity programs offered by the facility and that they are knowingly accepting full responsibility for their decision to participate in those activities and are releasing the facility from any and all responsibility for their participation. A waiver is a legal document that, by voluntarily signing, members and users give up, or waive, their right to institute a claim or litigation. These documents, when properly drafted and executed, are enforceable in most states. The waivers, however appropriate and legal, do not necessarily bar a user from filing a claim or from the possibility of litigation if the plaintiff's attorney advises that there is a viable cause of action. Thus, facilities must practice due diligence in the safe delivery of services in accordance with applicable standards and guidelines. An assumption of risk or waiver should be prepared by an attorney and should address the following at a minimum:

- The facility's programs and services to which the member or user has access and might use to pursue a program of physical activity
- The risks involved in participating in any moderate or more intense exercise, including the risk of a cardiac event or even death
- A statement that the member or user is aware of the risks involved, that the facility has explained those risks thoroughly, and that the user is willing to accept those risks
- The member's or user's willingness to accept all responsibility for participation in light of the information he or she has been provided and that the member or user is accepting complete responsibility for his or her actions and is releasing the facility from any and all liability associated with the decision, including the facility's ordinary negligence

The use of a waiver should be regular practice for all facilities. Ideally, all members and users should complete and sign a waiver form upon joining a facility. Both previous editions of *ACSM's Health/Fitness Facility Standards and Guidelines* and the 1998 IHRSA Health and Safety Standards indicate that the use of waivers should be a standard practice for health/fitness facility operators.

Risk management and emergency policies guideline 4. Facilities should have an incident report system for written documentation of all incidents that occur within the facility or within the facility's scope of responsibility. Such reports should be completed in a timely fashion and maintained on file, according to the statue of limitations for the government district in which they do business.

Facilities that desire to reduce their liability and provide their staff, members, and users with a safer work and physical activity environment should make the use of a written incident report system a part of their daily operating practice. An incident report system provides a means for the facility to document all incidents that involve individuals within the facility (e.g., staff, members and users, independent contractors).

A properly completed written document of an incident, whether it be a minor slip and fall or a major medical emergency, allows the facility to obtain information that can assist in the response to the incident and serves as a resource for any future requests for information about the incident. The information collected in an incident report becomes privileged information that can be released only to the proper authorities after approval of the involved parties. A proper incident report system should incorporate a written report that is completed by a qualified and responsible facility employee. Ideally, this report should be completed as soon as possible after an incident has occurred. The incident report system might include the following:

- Written incident report form (see forms 20 and 32 in appendix B for sample forms). The completed form should contain the following types of information:
  - Day, date, and time of the incident
  - Location of the incident
  - Person(s) involved in the incident
  - Witnesses to the incident
  - Staff responding to the incident
  - Actions taken in responding to the incident
  - Outcomes of the incident
- A team review of the incident should be conducted by qualified staff. The day after an incident occurs, it is advisable for the involved responders to review the report and resulting actions with facility management to assess the facility's response and to determine if further actions need to be taken.
- In the event of a major incident, the incident report should be forwarded to the facility's insurance carrier.
- It is always advisable for management to follow up with the involved parties to address any outstanding issues and make sure that the situation has been handled appropriately.

5

Professional Staff and Independent Contractors

The fitness and health club industry is a people-intensive industry. As such, several recent surveys indicate that many health/fitness facilities allocate upward of 40% of their gross revenues to wages and salaries. Not surprisingly, when a business allocates 40% or more of its resources to one specific factor, that area takes on critical importance to the success of that organization. The health and fitness industry is no different. Employees and independent contractors help to create and sustain the experiences that individuals undergo as a result of their membership in a particular health/fitness facility. Consequently, the employees and independent contractors in the industry have both a direct and an indirect effect on a health/fitness facility's level of operating success. Among the most critical of these employee and independent-contractor groups are the fitness and healthcare professionals who provide guidance, personal and group instruction, and supervision for facility users.

The most important role that staff and independent contractors who serve in the industry as fitness and healthcare professionals have is to ensure that a health/fitness facility's members' and users' experiences involving that facility are positive, including everything that should be done and could reasonably be done to ensure that members and users are exposed to the enumerable benefits of being physically active. Furthermore, these professionals also have responsibility for providing a physical activity environment within a health/fitness facility that is

reasonably safe. This responsibility includes the ability to respond to potential health-related emergencies.

Accordingly, fitness and healthcare professionals must have the necessary competencies for fulfilling their various roles and responsibilities. These competencies normally involve some combination of education, training, certification, and hands-on experience. Among fitness and healthcare professionals who are most likely to interact with facility members and users on a regular basis, help oversee essential program offerings, and assume supervisory responsibility for key initiatives within the facility are the fitness directors, fitness instructors, personal trainers, group exercise instructors, physical activity instructors, and lifestyle counselors. In addition to the aforementioned group of fitness and healthcare professionals, other key employees and independent contractors are the medical and healthcare liaisons, such as physical therapists, chiropractors, and physicians, who may interact directly or indirectly with the health/fitness facility members and users during the course of the physical activity programs being conducted.

This chapter presents standards and guidelines regarding the competency expectations for the aforementioned core group of professional staff and independent contractors. Table 5.1 provides a list of the three required standards for professional staff and independent contractors; tables 5.2 and 5.3 offer an overview of the combination of training (education, certification, and experience) that would constitute the reasonable expectation that a person would be competent to fulfill the professional demands of a particular position. Table 5.4 provides a list of the major professional certifications that are available in the health and fitness industry. Table 5.5 itemizes three recommended guidelines that health/fitness facilities should consider with regard to professional staff and independent contractors.

Standards for Health/ Fitness Facility Professional Staff and Independent Contractors

TABLE 5.1 Standards for Health/ Fitness Facility Professional Staff and Independent Contractors

1. The fitness and healthcare professionals who have supervisory responsibility for the physical activity programs (supervise and oversee members and users, staff, and independent contractors) of the facility must have an appropriate level of professional education, work experience, and/or certification.

2. The fitness and healthcare professionals who serve in counseling, instructional, and physical activity supervision roles for the facility must have an appropriate level of professional education, work experience, and/or certification.

3. Fitness and healthcare professionals engaged in prescribing, instructing, monitoring, or supervising of physical activity programs for facility members and users must have current automated external defibrillation and cardiopulmonary resuscitation (AED and CPR) certification from an organization qualified to provide such certification.

Professional staff and independent contractors standard 1. The fitness and healthcare professionals who have supervisory responsibility for the physical activity programs (supervise and oversee members and users, staff, and independent contractors) of the facility must have an appropriate level of pro-

fessional education, work experience, and/or certification.

The primary fitness and healthcare professionals who serve in a supervisory role are the fitness director, group exercise director, aquatics director, and program director. Table 5.2 provides examples of what might be considered an appropriate blend of professional education, certification, and work experience for some of the primary supervisory positions within the health and fitness industry.

Professional staff and independent contractors standard 2. The fitness and healthcare professionals who serve in counseling, instructional, and physical activity supervision roles for the facility must have an appropriate level of professional education, work experience, and/or certification.

The primary professional staff and independent contractors who serve in these roles are fitness instructors, group exercise instructors, lifestyle counselors, and personal trainers. Table 5.3 details examples of what might be considered the appropriate blend of professional education, certification, and work experience for some of the relevant positions in the health and fitness industry. Table 5.4 offers an overview of some of the major certifications available to these professionals in the health and fitness industry.

Professional staff and independent contractor standard 3. Fitness and healthcare professionals engaged in prescribing, instructing, monitoring, or supervising of physical activity programs for facility members and users must have current automated external defibrillation and cardiopulmonary resuscitation (AED and CPR) certification from an organization qualified to provide such certification.

Although the majority of fitness and healthcare professionals working in a fitness facility environment will never need to respond to a life-threatening cardiovascular event, the ability to respond in a competent manner is at the core of providing members and users with a reasonably safe physical activity environment. In its 2000 publication, *Guidelines for CPR and ECC*, the American Heart Association clearly indicates that those responding to a sudden cardiac event must be certified in AED and CPR.

TABLE 5.2 Recommended Competency Criteria for Program Supervisors in the Health and Fitness Industry

Professional position	Professional education	Professional certification	Professional experience
Aquatics director	4-year degree in fitness, exercise science, or related field from an accredited college or university is recommended, but not required.	Certification in advanced lifesaving and water safety from a nationally recognized organization is recommended. Certification as a pool operator from either a national (NSPI) or local organization or governmental agency is recommended.	Minimum of 3 years' experience as a lifeguard, water safety instructor, or swim instructor is recommended.
Fitness director	4-year degree in fitness or health-related field from an accredited college or university.	Fitness instructor or personal trainer certification from nationally recognized and accredited* certifying organization.	Minimum of 3 years' experience as a fitness professional working in the fitness and health industry in a health/fitness facility is recommended.
Group exercise director	2 years post-high school education in fitness, health, recreation, or related field from an accredited college or university is recommended but not required.	Group exercise instructor certification from a nationally recognized and accredited* certifying organization.	Minimum of 3 years' experience as a group exercise instructor working in the fitness and health industry in a health/fitness facility is recommended.
Program director	4-year degree in fitness, exercise science, or related field is recommended but not required.	Certification in fitness, group exercise, or related recreational field from a nationally recognized and accredited certifying organization is recommended.	Minimum of 3 years' experience working as an instructor or supervisor of physical activity or recreation programs is recommended.

* In this instance, the term *accredited* refers to certification programs that have received third-party approval of its certification procedures and practices from an appropriate agency, such as the National Commission for Certifying Agencies (NCCA).

TABLE 5.3 Recommended Competency Criteria for Instructors, Counselors, and Personal Trainers in the Health and Fitness Industry

Professional position	Professional education	Professional certification	Professional experience
Fitness instructor	4-year degree in fitness, exercise science, or related field recommended; with two years of college education in the field as a recommended minimum.	Fitness instructor or personal trainer certification from a nationally recognized and accredited* certifying organization.	Minimum of six months' experience working as a fitness instructor or personal trainer preferred.
Group exercise instructor	High school education required and two years of college education in fitness, exercise science, dance, or related field recommended but not required.	Group exercise instructor or leader certification from a nationally recognized and accredited* certifying organization.	Minimum of 100 hours' experience observing and teaching group exercise or fitness classes preferred.
Lifestyle counselor	4-year degree in fitness, health, or related field.	Fitness instructor or personal trainer certification from a nationally recognized and accredited certifying agency required. Additional certification from such organizations in lifestyle management, behavior change, or similar area recommended.	Minimum of one year's experience working as a fitness instructor or personal trainer, with at least 100 hours' experience in lifestyle counseling recommended but not required.

(continued)

TABLE 5.3 *(continued)*

Professional position	Professional education	Professional certification	Professional experience
Personal trainer	4-year degree in fitness, exercise science, or related field recommended; two years of college education in the field recommended but not required.	Fitness instructor or personal trainer certification from a nationally recognized and accredited certifying organization required.	Minimum of six months' experience working as a fitness instructor or personal trainer preferred.

*In this instance, the term *accredited* refers to certification programs that have received third-party approval of its certification procedures and practices from an appropriate agency, such as the National Commission for Certifying Agencies (NCCA).

TABLE 5.4 Major Certifications Available in the Health and Fitness Industry

Organization	Sample certifications	Examples of continuing education approach
American Council on Exercise	Group fitness, personal trainer, lifestyle and weight management consultant, clinical exercise specialist	Offers workshops, has CEC* providers and magazine and newsletter articles.
American College of Sports Medicine	Health fitness instructor, personal trainer, exercise specialist, clinical exercise physiologist	Offers workshops, national conferences, magazines, and CEC providers.
Aerobic and Fitness Association of America	Primary group exercise, personal fitness trainer, fitness practitioner	Offers workshops and has CEC providers.
East Coast Alliance	None	Offers workshops that promote CECs for most major certifying organizations.
International Dance Exercise Association	None	Offers national conference, workshops, and magazines and provides CECs for most major certifying organizations.
National Strength and Conditioning Association	Certified strength and conditioning specialist, personal trainer	Offers national and regional conferences and magazines and has CEC providers.
National Academy of Sports Medicine	Personal trainer, group trainer, performance-enhancement specialist	Offers workshops and has CEC providers.

*Continuing education credits (CEC)

Guidelines for Health/ Fitness Facility Professional Staff and Independent Contractors

TABLE 5.5 Guidelines for Health/ Fitness Facility Professional Staff and Independent Contractors

1. A facility that delivers or prescribes physical activity programs primarily or exclusively to members and users who are considered at an elevated risk for incurring a health-related problem because of their participation in physical activity (e.g., users over the age of 50 or those with coronary risk factors, diabetes, or clinical obesity) should have a medical liaison or medical advisory committee that assists in reviewing physical activity screening and programming protocols as well as emergency response protocols.

2. Facilities should provide the appropriate level of supervision and monitoring for each of the physical activity areas in the facility.

3. A facility should extend to each employee on staff the opportunity to receive training and certification in first aid and use of CPR and AED.

Professional staff and independent contractors guideline 1. A facility that delivers or prescribes physical activity programs primarily or exclusively to members and users considered at an elevated risk for incurring a health-related problem because of their participation in physical activity (e.g., users over the age of 50 or those with coronary risk factors, diabetes, or clinical obesity) should have a medical liaison or medical advisory committee that assists in reviewing physical activity screening and programming protocols as well as emergency response protocols.

Over the past decade, health/fitness facilities have seen a sharp rise in the number of members and users who are either over the age of 50 or who have one or more health-related disorders (e.g., cardiovascular disease, diabetes). These users are sometimes classified as *special populations.* The presence of a medical liaison or medical committee can assist a facility in ensuring that the protocols that the facility employs provide a reasonably safe physical activity experience for these special populations. If a medical liaison is considered, that individual should be a licensed physician. If a medical advisory committee is considered, the committee should include licensed physicians from various specialties as well as allied medical and healthcare professionals (e.g., nurse, physician's assistant, dietitian, emergency medical technician, chiropractor, podiatrist).

Professional staff and independent contractor guideline 2. Facilities should provide the appropriate level of supervision and monitoring for each of the physical activity areas in the facility.

The level of supervision and monitoring a facility provides for each of its physical activity areas is highly dependent on the facility's operating model and the level of risk that exists within each physical activity area. Because the health and fitness industry involves a variety of operating models (including facilities that are unstaffed, facilities that are staffed by one person, and facilities that may have as many as hundreds of employees and independent contractors), the ways in which physical activity areas are supervised and monitored can vary greatly. When staff or independent contractors are on duty, the facility should make every effort to supervise and monitor those physical activity areas that expose the members or users to the greatest risk. The following list details some of the physical activity areas that can expose the facility members or users to a heightened risk of cardiovascular, orthopedic, or musculoskeletal complications. Accordingly, these areas should be monitored or supervised on a regular basis if such scrutiny is consistent with the operating model of the facility.

- Cardiovascular equipment area
- Free weight equipment area
- Resistance equipment area
- Group exercise studios
- Tennis courts
- Basketball courts
- Racquet courts
- Pool, sauna, steam room, and whirlpool

Professional staff and independent contractor guideline 3. A facility should extend to each employee on staff the opportunity to receive training and certification in first aid and use of CPR and AED.

In the health and fitness industry, most fitness and healthcare professionals, as a rule, have AED and CPR certification. On occasion, however, some professionals do not. Accordingly, a health/fitness facility should always take steps to ensure that at least one person is on duty at all times when the facility is open who has the training and certification to administer first aid, CPR and/or AED. Because the first responders to many of the emergencies that occur in a health/fitness facility may not be fitness professionals, but instead are frontline, non-fitness professional staff, facilities should consider providing every employee the opportunity to be properly trained in both first aid and AED/CPR. It is in everyone's best interests for a health/fitness facility to give its employees the opportunity to be properly trained in these essential emergency practices. The more employees who receive this training, the greater the likelihood that the facility will be able to respond to emergencies in a timely and appropriate manner.

FOOTNOTE

The intent of this chapter is to provide the standards and guidelines that apply to the professional staff and independent contractors of a health/fitness facility. At the same time, it should be noted that according to IHRSA data, there are more than 50 different staff and independent contractor positions in the health and fitness industry, ranging from nonexempt hourly staff (such as housecleaning and front desk) to salaried exempt staff (such as membership directors and managers). Individuals who may hold one of these positions in a health/fitness facility, while not directly involved in the delivery of physical activity programs to facility users, still have a responsibility, when on duty, to provide the safest possible environment for the facility members and users.

Health/Fitness Facility Design and Construction

According to research sponsored by the International Health, Racquet and Sportclub Association (IHRSA), consumers weigh a facility's equipment and space offerings as one of the primary factors affecting their decision to join a club. According to IHRSA studies, facilities can be separated into two basic types: fitness-only facilities and multipurpose facilities. While these two broad categories provide a basis for identifying the two primary types of health/fitness facilities, each of these two categories can be further separated into subcategories, based on the type of business operation within a particular facility.

Fitness-only facilities are defined as facilities that offer space specifically for the pursuit of fitness activities. Typically, these facilities consist of areas for cardiovascular equipment, variable-resistance and selectorized circuit equipment, and free weight equipment. These facilities also include several common spaces, such as locker rooms and reception areas. In some cases, they include group exercise studios. According to data provided by IHRSA (2001 Profiles of Success), the average fitness-only facility is 32,402 sq ft (9,876 sq m). Sizewise, the smallest 25% of fitness-only clubs average approximately 13,000 sq ft (3,962 sq m), while the largest 25% average over 40,000 sq ft (12,192 sq m).

The major subcategories of fitness-only facilities are exercise studios, free weight gyms, apartment fitness areas, corporate fitness centers, and express facilities (such as Curves for Women). Exercise studios typically have one or two group exercise studios, a reception area, and locker rooms. Free weight gyms, on the other hand, normally provide a large free weight area, a reception area, and locker rooms. Fitness centers in apartment buildings and hotels generally are located in a somewhat limited space and typically feature a few pieces of cardiovascular, variable-resistance, and selectorized equipment. Corporate fitness centers range from small areas that contain a few pieces of variable-resistance, selectorized, and cardiovascular equipment to larger spaces that hold complete lines of cardiovascular, variable-resistance, and selectorized equipment. In fact, many of the smallest fitness-only facilities often occupy less than 3,000 sq ft (914 sq m) of space.

Multipurpose facilities are defined as facilities that offer both fitness facilities and one or more recreational spaces, such as racquet courts, pools, gymnasiums, spas, and outdoor recreational areas. According to a survey conducted by IHRSA (2004 Profiles of Success), the average multipurpose facility is 70,368 sq ft (21,448 sq m). Sizewise, the smallest 25% of this type of facility average 29,250 sq ft (8,915 sq m), while the largest 25% of this type of facility average over 99,000 sq ft (30,175 sq m). The majority of multipurpose facilities range in size from 40,000 to 100,000 sq ft (12,192 to 30,480 sq m).

The various subcategories of multipurpose health/fitness facilities include racquet courts only, pools only, gymnasiums only, facilities with tennis courts, and facilities with a blend of several activity areas. As a rule, almost all multipurpose facilities have fitness areas, racquet courts, and a gymnasium at a minimum. Pools and tennis courts are less common features for most multipurpose clubs. Some multipurpose facilities also have outdoor facilities, such as outdoor pools, ball fields, and even team-building venues. The largest multipurpose clubs tend to be those that have tennis facilities, gymnasiums, and outdoor facilities. More often than not, multipurpose facilities tend to be located in suburban settings because of the space demands of such facilities and the lower cost of available land.

Health/fitness facilities come in an array of sizes, shapes, and designs. Some are quite large, while others are considerably smaller. Some conduct their operations on a single floor, while others occupy multiple floors. Some have a bland appearance externally as well as internally, while others feature a design concept that emphasizes a more polished, "high-end" look.

Regardless of how large a facility is or how it looks, the key issue for a health/fitness facility is whether it is able to serve its intended and actual audience safely and effectively. This chapter addresses the factors in design and construction that can have a major impact on the ability of a health/fitness facility to provide a safe physical activity environment for its members and users.

Design and construction factors can be influenced by a number of considerations, including existing laws and regulations, architectural vision, available resources, and the activities and programs that are offered within a given facility. While some of these considerations are absolute in nature, others are not. For example, a facility's program offerings and certain design factors often go hand in hand. On one hand, the program offerings that are planned for a particular facility can have an influence on many of the decisions that are made concerning the design of a facility. On the other hand, the existing layout or space limitations within a given facility can help dictate (to a degree) what activity offerings are planned for that facility. Nonetheless, a health/fitness facility's program offerings typically play a key role in the level of success achieved by that facility.

This chapter presents standards and guidelines on health/fitness facility design and construction as they pertain to helping promote a safe physical-activity environment for facility users. Table 6.1 details the two required standards in this regard, whereas table 6.2 lists the 10 recommended guidelines for health/fitness facility design and construction. This chapter is not intended as a comprehen-

sive resource on health/fitness facility design and construction factors, but rather as a basic template for the design and construction features that are necessary for providing a reasonably safe physical activity environment.

Standards for Health/ Fitness Facility Design and Construction

TABLE 6.1 Standards for Health/ Fitness Facility Design and Construction

1. Facilities, to the extent required by law, must adhere to the standards of building design that relate to the designing, building, expanding, or renovating of space as presented by the Americans with Disabilities Act (ADA).
2. Facilities must be in compliance with all federal, state, and local building codes.

Health/fitness facility design and construction standard 1. Facilities, to the extent required by law, must adhere to the standards of building design that relate to the designing, building, expanding, or renovating of space as presented by the Americans with Disabilities Act (ADA).

The ADA has established clear requirements for making facilities accessible to people with disabilities. In most instances, when a facility undergoes significant renovation or expansion or when a new facility is built, the ADA requires that the space be made accessible to people with disabilities. Depending on the extent of work being performed or the costs involved, there are instances in which a facility may be able to perform work without having to comply fully with the requirements of the ADA. The local building departments in most communities can assist facilities in obtaining a clearer understanding of the ADA requirements. Appendixes C and D provide additional details on accessibility requirements. Among the key elements that concern accessibility within a health/fitness facility are the following:

• **Elevation changes.** The ADA requires that any change in elevation in excess of 0.5 in. (1.3 cm) must have a ramp or lift with a slope of 12 in. (30 cm) for every inch in elevation change. A mechanical lift or elevator can be used in place of a ramp in cases of extreme changes in height.

• **Passageway width.** The ADA requires that doors, entryways, and exits have a width of at least 36 in. (91 cm) to accommodate wheelchair access. In addition, hallways and circulation passages need to have a width of at least 60 in. (152 cm).

• **Height of switches and fountains.** The ADA requires that all light switches, water fountains, fire extinguishers, and AED devices be at a height that can be reached by a user in a wheelchair.

• **Signage.** The ADA expects facilities to provide essential signage that can be viewed by those who are visually impaired, particularly signage on emergency exits and signage that points out other key space locations.

• **Clear floor space.** The ADA requires that each piece of equipment have an adjacent clear floor space of at least 30 in. by 48 in. (76 cm by 122 cm).

Health/fitness facility design and construction standard 2. Facilities must be in compliance with all federal, state, and local building codes.

While federal requirements are consistent from one municipality to another, local building codes can vary drastically. It is imperative that facility operators be aware of the building codes in their community.

Guidelines for Health/ Fitness Facility Design and Construction

TABLE 6.2 Guidelines for Health/ Fitness Facility Design and Construction

1. Facilities should allocate sufficient space for physical activity zones so that defined circulation routes are adjacent to, rather than through, the physical activity areas.

2. Facilities should provide open-access circulation, which avoids blind corners, unnecessary doors, pointless partitions, and other hazards that would present a safety risk to members and users.

3. Facilities should separate physical activity spaces from operational, storage, and maintenance spaces.

4. Facilities should design both physical activity spaces and nonactivity spaces to provide sufficient space to accommodate the expected user demand placed on each space within the facility.

5. Facilities should provide all physical activity spaces with sufficient air circulation and fresh makeup air (i.e., outside air), which will allow the facility to maintain air quality, room temperatures, and humidity at safe and comfortable levels during times of physical activity.

6. Facilities should properly illuminate all facility spaces in order to allow members and users to safely navigate the various facility spaces and perform their physical activity regimens. Minimum safe illumination levels vary according to activity and should be carefully researched. The emerging need for energy conservation requires lighting solutions that take advantage of the available daylighting sources, automatic control devices, and the latest technologies in lamp and fixture design.

7. Facilities should be designed to maintain background noise levels below 70 decibels and never above 90 decibels. Sound transmission through defining perimeter partitions of a noise-generating activity area should be limited to a level that does not adversely affect the functionality of neighboring spaces.

8. Floor surfaces in physical activity areas should provide the proper level of absorption and slip resistance to minimize the risk of users' incurring impact or fall-related injuries.

9. Facilities should have wall surfaces in activity spaces that are nonabrasive, flush, and free of protrusions that could cause impact injuries. Activity spaces that involve airborne projectiles, such as volleyballs or basketballs, should have a perimeter ball-containment barrier to protect users in adjacent areas and walkways.

10. When physical activity spaces have depth and distance parameters that can affect an individual's safety, then the facility should provide the appropriate markings to ensure that users are aware of these depth and distance parameters.

Health/fitness facility design and construction guideline 1. Facilities should allocate sufficient space for physical activity zones so that defined circulation routes are adjacent to rather than through the physical activity areas.

Circulation areas are spaces that allow users to enter, exit, and transverse the various physical activity zones. These circulation spaces should provide pathways that accommodate access to each area,* including the functional spaces in and around exercise equipment. To this end, the pathways should be at least 36 in. (91 cm) across and be located adjacent to the physical activity areas so that users do not have to pass directly through a physical activity area to access another area.

Note: The ADA requires that one piece of each type of exercise equipment have a clear floor space equal to 30 in. by 48 in. (76 cm by 122 cm) and be served by an accessible route.

Health/fitness facility design and construction guideline 2. Facilities should provide open-access circulation, which avoids blind corners, unnecessary doors, pointless partitions, and other hazards that would present a safety risk to members and users.

Open circulation refers to spaces that provide adequate sight lines and reduce or eliminate the possibility of members' and users' quickly encountering hazardous situations. The following are some of the steps that a facility can take to provide open circulation:

• **Avoid blind corners in two-way circulation areas.** This objective can be accomplished in several ways, including soft corners, low walls at intersections, mirrors, and appropriate warning signage.

• **Avoid the use of doors that open up into circulation paths and hallways.** When doors are mandated by local codes or privacy situations, providing proper warning signage can help reduce any risk presented by these door locations.

• **Provide circulation areas that, by the nature of their design, communicate a path of safe passage.**

Health/fitness facility design and construction guideline 3. Facilities should separate physical activity spaces from operational, storage, and maintenance spaces.

By separating back-of-the house operational spaces from physical activity spaces designed to be used by members and users, the facility can reduce or eliminate the likelihood that members and users will enter a facility area that would immediately expose them to an increased safety risk from items such as cleaning supplies, maintenance equipment, and related materials. The following are examples of back-of-the house operational areas that should be separated from the physical activity areas:

• **Laundry.** This area normally contains cleaning agents that, according to OSHA, present an increased risk of exposure to hazardous chemicals.

• **Equipment rooms for pools and whirlpools.** These areas commonly house chemicals and other agents that may be harmful, especially if inhaled directly.

• **Maintenance rooms.** These rooms commonly contain equipment (such as saws, chemical supplies, and power tools) that could accidentally cause harm to a facility member or user.

• **Mechanical and electrical rooms.** These rooms contain equipment that could expose members and users directly or indirectly to dangerous situations, such as exposed wires, high temperatures, and dangerous gases.

Health/fitness facility design and construction guideline 4. Facilities should design both physical activity spaces and nonactivity spaces to provide sufficient space to accommodate the expected user demand placed on each space within the facility.

In designing a fitness facility, one of the most critical factors in providing a safe physical activity environment is to make sure that there is the appropriate amount of square footage to allow for the unencumbered use of the facility by each member or user while that individual is in the facility. While no industry-established standard currently exists for the appropriate space allocation per member or user in a facility, the following industry averages, based on IHRSA-derived data, are recommended:

• Fitness-only type facilities should provide approximately 12 sq ft (3.7 sq m) per membership, depending on the facility's business model and target audience. The amount of space allocated per membership may range from as low as 5 sq ft (1.5 sq m) per member to as high as 30 sq ft (9 sq m) per member.

- Multipurpose-type facilities should provide approximately 27 sq ft (7.2 sq m) per member. A space allocation that depends on the target audience, the facility's program offerings, and the facility's business model could range from as low as 10 sq ft (3 sq m) per member to as high as 50 sq ft (15 sq m) per member.

- Group exercise rooms or studios should provide between 40 and 60 sq ft (12 and 18 sq m) per expected member or user in the space at any given time.

- The fitness floor should provide between 25 and 50 sq ft (7.6 and 15.2 sq m) per piece of equipment on the floor and space for stretching that allows 40 to 60 sq ft (12 to 18 sq m) of space per member or user. Furthermore, an allowance of 10% to 15% additional space should be allocated for circulation.

Health/fitness facility design and construction guideline 5. Facilities should provide all physical activity spaces with sufficient air circulation and fresh makeup air (i.e., outside air), which will allow the facility to maintain air quality, room temperatures, and humidity at safe and comfortable levels during times of physical activity.

Air circulation is one of the most critical elements when designing and operating a health/fitness facility. When a room is filled with members and users exercising at a moderate to high intensity, the heat and humidity load increases dramatically. This can place an increased level of heat stress on the members and users and may result in dehydration, heat exhaustion, heatstroke, or (in rare instances) cardiovascular emergencies. In addition to the increased heat load that can result from improper air circulation, a risk of poor air quality exists that can expose members and users to airborne pathogens that can increase the risk of respiratory disorders or other airborne illnesses. Facilities can provide sufficient air circulation by taking into consideration the following factors:

- **Maintain relative humidity at 60% or lower in all physical activity spaces.** Ideally, a relative humidity level of 50% or lower is the desired goal, but maintaining levels below 60% is necessary.

- **Maintain air temperature for all physical activity areas between 68 and 72 °F or 20 and 23 °C.** The key is to maintain these temperature ranges, whether the room is empty or fully occupied by members and users who are engaging in moder-

ate to vigorous physical activity. This guideline refers to the fact that the heating, ventilation, and air conditioning (HVAC) system within the facility should have the capability to adjust airflow to meet the demands of each space. Ideally, a facility should establish specific HVAC zones that allow each zone to provide airflow to areas of similar heat stress. Examples of establishing similar circulation zones include group activity studios on one zone, the fitness floor on one zone, racquet courts on one zone, locker rooms on one zone, and pools and wet areas on one zone.

- **Ensure that wet areas, such as shower areas, steam rooms, whirlpool areas, and swimming pools, have negative exhaust (more exhausted air than vented air).** Negative air allows air to be pulled through and out of these areas rather than stagnating in those areas.

- **Make sure that the entire HVAC system is balanced and provides air circulation at the proper cubic feet per minute (CFM) in each of the respective physical activity areas.** CFM is a quantitative measure that can be used to indicate the amount of airflow that is moved through a vent. The CFM for physical activity areas will vary based on the heat load to which the area is exposed. For example, rooms, such as group exercise studios, will require higher CFM than racquet courts. Likewise, the cardiovascular equipment area will require higher CFM than the free weight area. Facilities should consider hiring a qualified mechanical engineer to provide the guidance and assistance that might be required in this regard.

- **Keep the mechanical system clean.** Most mechanical systems require that the vents be cleaned on a monthly basis and that the coils in the cooling system be cleaned on a quarterly basis. This preventive maintenance will allow the system to provide better air circulation and will also prevent the buildup of dirt and microbes in the system.

- **Make sure that there is an adequate mix of external fresh air and recirculated internal air moving through the facility.** The higher the percentage of external air, the less likely the chance that the system will circulate air that contains airborne pathogens that were released by those who use the facility. The minimum level of outside external air is 10%, with a goal of getting as close to 50% as possible. Many office buildings in which facilities lease space contain almost 100% recirculated air, with no blending of external air.

Health/fitness facility design and construction guideline 6. Facilities should properly illuminate all facility spaces in order to allow members and users to safely navigate the various facility spaces and perform their physical activity regimens. Minimum safe illumination levels vary according to activity and should be carefully researched. The emerging need for energy conservation requires lighting solutions that take advantage of available daylighting sources, automatic control devices, and the latest technologies in lamp and fixture design.

Proper illumination is a necessity for a reasonably safe environment. The proper level of illumination can vary from space to space, depending on the activity being performed. Spaces in which physical activity requires fine hand-eye motor coordination (e.g., playing tennis) require a higher degree of illumination, compared with those facility areas (such as a yoga studio) where the need for lower levels of illumination might be appropriate. Another important factor regarding proper levels of illumination is that a facility's users must be able to read all signage and must have sufficient visual scan of the signage to be able to avoid hazardous situations. The following are among the more important considerations for illumination:

• **Light levels in the majority of physical activity spaces, as measured at eye level, should be at least 50 foot-candles.** In selected areas, such as a tennis court or racquet court, light levels approaching 70 foot-candles at eye level are preferred, while on a volleyball court at floor level, a foot-candle level of 50 is appropriate. Each activity area will have slightly different illumination requirements, based on the activity being performed.

• **When designing light sources, an effort should be made to use either natural light or artificial light sources that produce indirect soft lighting instead of direct lighting in an area.** Natural lighting can be emphasized by using windows with tinted and insulated glass. Indirect light sources that bounce light off walls, floors, or ceilings are preferred to direct light sources. The most-often-used artificial lighting sources include incandescent light fixtures with soft light bulbs, fluorescent light fixtures, metal-halide light fixtures (for racquet courts and gymnasiums), and mercury-vapor light fixtures (for racquet courts and gymnasiums).

• **Adjustable light sources (dimmer-switch controlled) should be provided, whenever possible, for areas such as group exercise studios,** massage rooms, mind–body activity areas, and similar spaces.

• **Light fixtures should be mounted at the appropriate height in order to ensure the proper level of illumination and the avoidance of members' and users' exposure to excessive heat or direct light.** In fitness areas, group exercise studios, and most other areas of the facility, ceiling-mounted lighting should be at least 8 ft (2.4 m) above the floor, while wall-mounted lighting should be above eye level. In gymnasiums, tennis courts, and other indoor spaces involving ball-based sports, all lighting fixtures should be mounted at a sufficient height where those fixtures cannot be damaged by those objects or people involved in the activity being performed. This means the fixtures should be located 20 to 30 ft (6.1 to 9.1 m) above floor level.

Health/fitness facility design and construction guideline 7. Facilities should be designed to maintain background noise levels below 70 decibels and never above 90 decibels. Sound transmission through defining perimeter partitions of a noise-generating activity area should be limited to a level that does not adversely affect the functionality of neighboring spaces.

A health/fitness facility can be a cauldron of sounds ranging from the background noise of members and users talking to the sound produced by audio systems. Background noise levels are measured in decibels. Levels of 90 decibels or greater, despite the circumstances, are too loud. Ongoing exposure of members and users and staff to decibel levels in excess of 90 can cause hearing damage. Some health and fitness spaces, such as group exercise studios and the fitness floor, will naturally have higher decibel levels, while spaces such as the mind–body studio or the massage room generally have much lower decibel levels. As a general rule, decibel levels in the range of 30 to 40 allow for most individuals to receive sound without being exposed to noise levels that can result in damage to their hearing. Among the factors that should be taken into consideration when attempting to limit excessive decibel levels in a health/fitness facility are the following:

• **Group exercise studios tend to generate the highest decibel levels (levels between 80 and 90 decibels are common).** To assist in reducing the sound levels in the spaces, facilities should provide ceiling, floor, and wall surfaces that allow for moderate sound absorption, adjust audio systems so sound levels cannot be raised above 90 decibels, and develop and enforce policies that ensure that the facility's instructors adhere to the recommended sound levels. In addition, these spaces should be designed with additional sound-absorption materials to prevent the movement of excess noise levels into adjacent spaces.

• **Spaces that are intended to provide low levels of sound (such as massage rooms, mind–body studios, and lounges) should be designed to have additional sound-absorbing materials in the ceilings, floors, and walls.**

Health/fitness facility design and construction guideline 8.
Floor surfaces in physical activity areas should provide the proper level of absorption and slip resistance to minimize the risk of users' incurring impact or fall-related injuries.

Some physical activity areas (such as the group exercise studio, basketball court, racquet courts, and fitness floor) house activities that can expose users to impact stresses. In many cases, the activities performed in these areas can more than double the forces to which a member's or user's body is exposed. Fortunately, through the proper design and installation of floor surfaces, many of these additional forces can be absorbed by the floor surface rather than by the individual's musculoskeletal system. The key point with regard to floor surfaces is that facilities should adhere to the Deutsches Institut fur Normung (DIN) standards when installing physical activity floor surfaces. According to the DIN standards, a floor must meet five criteria: shock absorption, standard vertical deflection, deflective-indentation sliding characteristics, ball reflection, and rolling load. Each of these five characteristics can be used to help evaluate the suitability of a floor for specific physical activity functions, including the following:

• **Sport function.** These are floors that serve a recreational or performance sport function, such as a basketball court or racquetball court. These court floors need to provide good surface friction and ball reflection. In deciding which floors to use for this purpose, it is critical to employ a consistent subfloor that absorbs impact equally at all points on the floor and generates minimal deflective indentation. In addition, these floors should provide a moderate level of surface friction that balances the ability to gain traction with the ability for sliding. These floors normally have a subfloor system (consisting of fur-

ring strips and shock-absorbing materials) that is covered by a solid wood surface or rubber surface that allows for sliding movement.

• **Protective function.** The primary role served by these floors is the reduction of chronic-impact injuries or acute-impact injuries, such as those that could occur in a group exercise studio. These floors should have outstanding shock absorption, little vertical deformation, and sliding characteristics. Normally, these floors have a three-layer system consisting of a bottom shock-absorbing layer (neoprene shock pads, rubber pads, springs), a middle layer that has two layers of plywood, and a top layer consisting of a wood or rubber surface.

• **Material–technical function.** These floors, which should meet criteria for both sport and protective function, are excellent for facilities that use space for multiple activities, such as a basketball court that also serves as a group exercise space. According to the DIN standards, this type of floor should have the following characteristics:

Shock absorption	53% minimum
Vertical deformation	2.3 mm minimum
Deflective indentation	15% maximum
Sliding characteristic	.5 to .7 range
Ball deflection	90% minimum
Rolling load	337.6 lb (153.1 kg)

Facility operators should discuss their facility's requirements with the floor manufacturers to ensure that the floors that they select for their facility are constructed in accordance with DIN standards.

Health/fitness facility design and construction guideline 9.
Facilities should have wall surfaces in activity spaces that are nonabrasive, flush, and free of protrusions that could cause impact injuries. Activity spaces that involve airborne projectiles, such as volleyballs and basketballs, should have a perimeter ball-containment barrier to protect individuals in adjacent areas and walkways.

Health/fitness facility design and construction guideline 10.
When physical activity spaces have depth and distance parameters that can affect an individual's safety, then the facility should provide the appropriate markings to ensure that users are aware of these depth and distance parameters.

Physical activity areas that can pose an increased risk to members and users (because of either depth or distance factors) include the pool, basketball court, and racquet courts. In this regard, the following recommendations apply:

• **Pools.** Pools present the greatest risk to member and user safety caused by the presence of water and changes in depth. Facilities should follow parameters of the National Pool and Spa Institute (NPSI) for marking pool depths and distances, subject to local and state codes. Pools are expected to provide proper depth markings at various points, especially when there are changes in pool depth.

• **Basketball courts and racquetball courts.** These courts have specific markings and dimensions established by the respective sport governing bodies. Facilities should ensure that these recommendations are followed in the design and installation of the courts.

Additional details on specific design or construction parameters for health/fitness facilities are presented in appendix A.

CHAPTER

Health/Fitness
Facility Equipment

According to industry research, the average health/fitness facility spends about $15 to $25 (U.S.) per square foot on equipment before opening its doors to the public for the first time. This relatively large investment indicates the important role that equipment plays in providing facility users with the opportunity to pursue their physical activity interests and needs. This initial investment in equipment is further compounded by the need for facility owners to reinvest in equipment on an annual basis to stay current with equipment trends (function and safety) and to deal with the depreciation and inevitable wear on equipment. The basic categories of fitness equipment that play the most significant role in the industry when it comes to delivering physical activity programs are cardiovascular equipment, variable-resistance equipment, free weight equipment, and fitness sport accessory equipment.

- **Cardiovascular equipment.** Cardiovascular equipment exists in 86% of health/fitness facilities and is second only to free weight equipment in terms of its presence. According to International Health, Racquet and Sportclub Association (IHRSA), cardiovascular equipment areas were the number one expansion priority for facility operators in 2004. Although cardiovascular equipment has been in existence for almost as long as the health and fitness industry has been in existence, over the last 15 years, it has taken on an escalating level of importance in the marketing and programming of health/fitness facilities.

- **Variable-resistance and selectorized equipment.** According to statistics provided by IHRSA for 2004, variable-resistance and selectorized equipment can be found in more than 80% of all clubs.

Selectorized resistance equipment is strength training equipment that uses weight stacks and pulley mechanisms to provide resistance. The advantage of this type of resistance exercise is that it provides a safe and time-efficient method of strength training, one that often has particular appeal for the average health/fitness facility member or user. Variable resistance equipment is quite similar to selectorized resistance equipment except that it employs a device (usually a cam) that allows the level of resistance provided to the exercises at any given point in time to vary according to predetermined strength curve of the muscles involved in the exercise.

- **Free weight equipment.** Free weight equipment has been in existence longer than any other form of exercise equipment. According to a survey conducted for IHRSA in 2004, 95% of clubs indicate that they offer free weight equipment. These statistics indicate that free weight equipment is currently the most popular type of exercise equipment in the health and fitness club industry.

- **Fitness sport accessory equipment.** Fitness sport accessory equipment includes Pilates gear, bands and tubes, fitness-testing apparatus, plyometric paraphernalia, medicine balls and exercise balls, foam rollers, and other devices that can assist individuals in achieving their health and fitness goals. Other accessories include equipment (such as weight training belts and protective lenses) that can be used to provide a safer environment for a facility's members and users as they engage in activities of their choosing.

This chapter presents standards and guidelines pertaining to equipment that is found in health/

fitness facilities. Table 7.1 details the one required standard on fitness equipment; table 7.2 lists the three recommended guidelines that health/fitness facilities should consider when acquiring fitness equipment. It should be noted that this chapter is not intended to provide an in-depth review of health and fitness equipment. In contrast, it is designed to offer information regarding equipment that health/fitness facilities can use in their efforts to provide a safe and productive physical activity environment for their members and users.

Standards for Health/ Fitness Facility Equipment

TABLE 7.1 Standards for Health/ Fitness Facility Equipment

1. The aquatic and pool facilities must provide the proper safety equipment and signage according to state and local codes and regulations.

Health/fitness facility equipment standard 1. The aquatic and pool facilities must provide the proper safety equipment and signage according to state and local codes and regulations.

State and local governments have specific requirements regarding the safety equipment that must be present in an aquatic area. Examples of the types of equipment that may be required include a spine board, a 25 ft (7.6 m) safety rope with a buoy, a shepherd's crook, lifejackets, a rescue tube, blankets, and a first-aid kit. If a facility has more than one aquatic venue, then each venue must have the proper equipment.

Guidelines for Health/ Fitness Facility Equipment

TABLE 7.2 Guidelines for Health/ Fitness Facility Equipment

1. Facilities should provide a sufficient quantity and quality of equipment so that the facility is able to fulfill its mission, purpose, and intended

function for its targeted members and users.
2. Facilities should have a preventive maintenance program for their fitness equipment, including documentation showing when the scheduled work was performed.
3. All physical activity areas should have a clock, a chart of target heart rates, and a chart depicting ratings of perceived exertion to enable members and users to monitor their level of physical exertion.

Health/fitness facility equipment guideline 1. Facilities should provide a sufficient quantity and quality of equipment so that the facility is able to adequately fulfill its mission, purpose, and intended function for its targeted members and users.

Health/fitness facilities vary considerably in their intended mission and purpose. For example, some facilities, such as multipurpose facilities, focus on serving the fitness and recreational needs of the family market, while some fitness-only clubs address the muscular strength and endurance interests of a young male population. In recent years, a substantial number of women-only facilities have opened; their basic business model involves providing a nonintimidating general fitness environment for their clients. Such diversity of missions and purposes has a significant impact on the variety, quantity, and quality of equipment that is made available to members and users.

Decisions concerning the kind of equipment to buy, how much equipment to buy, and how much to spend on equipment can be affected by a number of factors, which can vary from facility to facility. The following information can be used to help clarify the key issues pertaining to such discussions:

• **Cardiovascular equipment.** The second most popular category of equipment in the health and fitness industry, cardiovascular equipment, should potentially be part of every health/fitness facility. The most popular types of cardiovascular equipment include treadmills, elliptical trainers, rowing machines, stair climbers, bicycles, recumbent bicycles, upper-body ergometers, and total-body machines (e.g., cross-body trainers).

Over and above the business model and the target audience of a given facility, the quantity of cardiovascular equipment that a health/fitness facility acquires will depend on several variables, including the number of members and users, the usage patterns for each category of cardiovascular equipment, and member and user demographics. The minimum number of pieces of any one category should be two machines; the ideal quantity is dependent on the aforementioned variables.

While no precise criteria exist in the industry for determining the appropriate quantity or mix of cardiovascular equipment, common practice in the industry is to provide sufficient equipment to accommodate at least 25% of the individuals that are expected to use the facility during any given 2 h time period. For example, if a hypothetical facility has 2,000 members and users, then that facility is likely to see approximately 500 (or 25%) of those members on a daily basis. Furthermore, during any given two hour time period, it can expect to see no more than 33% of those daily users, or 165 users. If the criterion is one piece of cardiovascular equipment for every four members and users in a facility, then the facility in this example would need approximately 40 pieces of cardiovascular equipment.

• **Variable-resistance and selectorized equipment.** Variable-resistance and selectorized machines are designed to provide individuals with a relatively safe, time-efficient method to engage in strength exercise. Some of these machines have multiple stations that collectively offer a whole-body workout. Others address only a single muscle or area of the body. In those instances, a series of selectorized/variable-resistance machines will be required for achieving a complete strength training regimen. At a minimum, one machine for each major muscle group in the body will be required. Depending on the facility's professional focus, it is recommended that every health/fitness facility have at least one resistance circuit. At a minimum, facilities should make sure that they have sufficient machines to accommodate anticipated demand by its members and users for strength exercise. While no specific industry criteria exist in this regard, common practice within the health/fitness industry dictates that at least one circuit be provided for each 1,000 members and users.

• **Free weight equipment.** The most popular type of exercise equipment in health/fitness facilities is free weight equipment, which can include such items as dumbbells, barbells and plates, plate-loaded benches and machines, and benches and machines that can be used for performing exercises that employ barbells and dumbbells. The type and quantity of free weight equipment that a facility provides will depend on that facility's mem-

bership and usage patterns as well as its targeted audience.

• **Fitness accessory equipment.** Over the past 10 years, the interest in and the demand for functional and performance-based fitness training have grown tremendously. Types of fitness sport accessory equipment that can facilitate such functional and performance-based training include, but are not limited to, medicine balls, exercise balls, tubes and bands, foam rollers, Pilates-based equipment, plyometric benches, rope ladders, cones, and steps. The quantity of fitness sport accessory equipment that a facility acquires is highly dependent on the facility's member and user demographics, the number of facility members and users, and the qualifications of its staff and independent contractors.

• **Group exercise equipment.** Group exercise studios are one of the most highly used spaces in a health/fitness facility. The types of program offerings that are typically conducted in a group exercise facility include, but are not limited to, group cycling classes, stretching classes, low-impact classes, yoga classes, martial arts fitness classes, calisthenic classes, weight equipment–based classes, and sport performance classes. Because of the large variety of classes that can be offered within such areas, a facility should provide the equipment that is necessary to accommodate the needs of those classes. Selected ancillary equipment may include group cycles, exercise mats, step benches, tubes and bands, exercise balls, and medicine balls.

Health/fitness facility equipment guideline 2. Facilities should have a preventive maintenance program for their fitness equipment, including documentation showing when the scheduled work was performed.

Manufacturers of fitness equipment provide limited warranties on their equipment as well as recommendations for its ongoing care. The proper care of equipment is essential for several reasons. For example, failure to have and adhere to a preventive maintenance system will almost always lead to equipment breakdowns and a heightened risk to users' safety and the facility's subsequent exposure to litigation. In most instances, the preventive maintenance of fitness equipment is quite similar. Facilities, however, are encouraged to closely follow the manufacturer's recommendations for standard preventive maintenance. Tables 7.3 and 7.4 provide an overview of the most common preventive maintenance practices for

TABLE 7.3 Common Preventive Maintenance Practices for Resistance Training Equipment

Equipment	Daily care	Weekly care	Monthly care	As needed
Variable-resistance equipment	• Clean frames with mild soap and water. • Clean upholstery with mild soap and water.	• Check all cables and bolts and tighten as needed. • Check moving parts and adjust as needed.	Lubricate guide rods with lightweight oil.	• Repair or replace pads. • Replace cables if needed.
Free weight benches	• Clean frames with mild soap and water. • Clean upholstery with mild soap and water.	• Check all cables and bolts and tighten as needed. • Check moving parts and adjust as needed.		• Repair or replace pads. • Replace cables if needed.
Dumbbells and bars	Clean off bars with dry cloth.	Check all screws and bolts and tighten as needed.	Use lightweight oil on cloth to remove any rust.	Repair or replace broken bars and dumbbells.

TABLE 7.4 Common Preventive Maintenance Practices for Cardiovascular Equipment

Equipment	Daily care	Weekly care	Monthly care	As needed
Bicycles and recumbent bicycles	• Clean off control panel with damp cloth. • Clean off seats with mild soap and water. • Clean housing with mild soap and water.	• Check equipment diagnostics on control panel for any warnings or indications of problems. • Check all screws and bolts and tighten as needed. • If positioned on carpet, vacuum underneath.	Remove housing covering the bike and clean out any dust or lint.	Refer to manufacturer's guidelines.
Elliptical trainers and stair climbers	• Clean off control panel with damp cloth. • Clean housing and pedals with mild soap and water.	• Check equipment diagnostics on control panel for any warnings or indications of problems. • Check all screws and bolts and tighten as needed. • Vacuum.	Remove housing covering the elliptical or stair climber and clean out any dust or lint.	Refer to manufacturer's guidelines.
Treadmills	• Clean off control panel with damp cloth. • Clean housing and pedals with mild soap and water.	• Check equipment diagnostics on control panel for any warnings or indications of problems. • Check all screws and bolts and tighten as needed. • If positioned on carpet, vacuum underneath.	• Clean belts using a damp cloth. • Check belt and deck surface and lubricate as needed. • Check rollers and adjust if out of alignment.	• Replace belts if needed. • Replace deck surfaces if diagnostics indicate. • Refer to manufacturer's guidelines.

resistance training equipment and cardiovascular equipment, respectively.

Health/fitness facility equipment guideline 3. All physical activity areas should have a clock, a chart of target heart rates, and a chart depicting ratings of perceived exertion to enable members and users to monitor their level of physical exertion.

Having a clock and a target heart rate chart available in the various physical activity areas allows facility members and users to monitor their level of physical exertion and assists them in achieving their desired training intensity and duration. A rating of perceived exertion chart can be substituted for or used to complement a target heart rate chart as a means of providing individuals with an easy-to-understand method of monitoring their level of intensity of physical activity.

Health/Fitness Facility Operating Practices

Operating practices refer to those administrative policies, practices, procedures, and systems that a facility uses to deliver its products and services to members and users in a manner that is consistent with the vision and business model of the facility. Operating practices can range from the policies governing scheduling appointments to the practice of conducting orientations for new members. The more formalized these operating practices are, the more likely the facility will consistently deliver its products and services in the desired manner.

In the health and fitness industry, there are many excellent operating practices. As a result, no one best method for operating a health/fitness facility exists. Instead, there are benchmarks or best practices that clearly define the parameters of what health/fitness facility operators need to do in order to run their business successfully. The most successful facility operators tend to divide operations into two important components: operating standards and systems. Operating standards are the basic expectations that a facility has for delivering a specified practice. They serve as a framework for staff concerning the facility's mission statement. The systems are the tools that staff can use to meet the operational standards or expectations.

This chapter presents the standards and guidelines for a health/fitness facility's operating practices. Table 8.1 lists four standards for health/fitness facility operations. This chapter is not intended as an in-depth look at facility operations. In contrast, it is designed to provide a template regarding operational practices that health/fitness facilities can use as appropriate.

Table 8.4 lists the four recommended guidelines pertaining to operating practices of health/fitness facilities.

Standards for Health/ Fitness Facility Operating Practices

TABLE 8.1 Standards for Health/ Fitness Facility Operating Practices

1. Facilities must have a system in operation that monitors the entry to and usage of the facility by all individuals, including members and users.

2. Facilities that offer a sauna, steam room, or whirlpool must ensure that these areas are maintained at the proper temperature and that the appropriate warning systems are in place to notify members and users of any unacceptable risks and changes in temperature.

3. Facilities that offer members and users access to a pool or whirlpool ensure that the pool water chemistry is maintained in accordance with state and local codes.

4. A facility that offers youth services or programs must provide appropriate supervision.

Health/fitness facility operating practices standard 1. Facilities must have a system in operation that monitors the entry to and usage of the facility by all individuals, including members and users.

The ability to identify all individuals entering the facility and the members and users who are participating in the various physical activity programs offered by the facility is important for at least three reasons. First, by knowing who enters the facility, the staff members at the facility can enhance the level of safety in the facility by ensuring that only those with privileges have access to the facility. Second, by having a knowledge of which members and users are in the facility, the staff at the facility can respond more effectively to potential emergency situations. Third, having knowledge of who is using the facility at any given time can influence the development of staffing and supervision schedules for each area of the facility, which in turn can provide a safer physical activity environment for the members and users.

Monitoring systems can be either manual or computerized. Manual systems involve having members and users sign in whenever they enter the facility. With a manual system, most facilities expect the members and users not only to sign in but also to record the time of their entry. Computerized systems require that the members and users present an identification card to the facility that is used to record their visits. The computerized systems automatically record the time of a person's entry and maintain records of every visit.

Health/fitness facility operating practices standard 2. Facilities that offer a sauna, steam room, or whirlpool must ensure that these areas are maintained at the proper temperature and that the appropriate warning systems are in place to notify members and users of any unacceptable risks and changes in temperature.

Saunas, steam rooms, and whirlpools are all potentially high-risk areas to members and users because of the high temperature and humidity that are generated in these spaces. A facility's failure to maintain these three areas at what are considered safe temperatures can further expose members and users to harmful conditions such as hyperthermia, heat exhaustion, heatstroke, and cardiovascular emergencies. Even when maintained at the proper temperature, these three areas can still result in dangerous consequences if individuals are not warned of the associated risks and precautions that go with their use. Heart attack and stroke would be very rare. Orthostatic syncope (i.e., a condition where a person feels dizzy or faint from the venous pooling of blood that occurs upon changing from a supine to upright position) would be more likely. Table 8.2 provides an overview of the recommended temperature ranges and precautions in saunas, steam rooms, and whirlpool areas.

Health/fitness facility operating practices standard 3. Facilities that offer members and

---

TABLE 8.2   Recommended Temperatures and Precautions for Saunas, Steam Rooms, and Whirlpools

Wet area	Temperature range recommendations	Precautions
Sauna	160-170 °F (71-77 °C)	• Limit use to 10 minutes at one time. • Wait at least 10 minutes after exercise before entering. • If you are pregnant or have heart disease, kidney disease, and/or other medical conditions that might be adversely affected by high heat, do not use.
Steam room	100-110 °F (38-43 °C)	• Limit use to 10 minutes at one time. • Wait at least 10 minutes after exercise before entering. • If you are pregnant or have heart disease, kidney disease, and/or other medical conditions that might be adversely affected by high heat, do not use.
Whirlpool	102-105 °F (39-41 °C)	• Limit use to 10 minutes at one time. • Wait at least 10 minutes after exercise before entering. • If you are pregnant or have heart disease, kidney disease, and/or other medical conditions that might be adversely affected by high heat, do not use.

users access to a pool or whirlpool must ensure that the pool water chemistry is maintained in accordance with state and local codes.

In most states, either the state or local municipality with governing authority establishes standards for the proper water chemistry. Most state and local codes provide minimums for the various chemical levels of the water. Facility operators can also refer to the National Spa and Pool Institute (NSPI) for more thorough information on the proper water chemistry for pools and whirlpools (spas). Table 8.3 provides an overview of the ranges recommended by the NSPI for the most critical water chemical levels in a pool or whirlpool.

Health/fitness facility operating practices standard 4. A facility that offers youth services or programs must provide appropriate supervision.

Properly caring for and supervising any children who are present in a health/fitness facility are critical responsibilities. Accordingly, facilities that offer some form of children's programs or services must have in place systems that ensure that these designated practices are followed:

• **Medical history.** When a child is in the exclusive control of a facility (i.e., the parent or guardian is not in the facility), basic medical information must be obtained by the facility and available to the person in the facility who is responsible for the child. This requires that the facility staff work with the parents to collect relevant information, which should focus on any allergies, illnesses, and any other special medical conditions that the child may have.

• **Waiver and release.** Each parent or guardian must complete a waiver and release for the children whom they leave in the facility's care. In some states, parents and/or guardians cannot disclaim their responsibility or waive or release their children's rights; therefore, facility operators should check the relevant laws in their state.

• **Sign-in and sign-out.** A facility must have an appropriate system for ensuring that children are dropped off and picked up by authorized individuals. An appropriate record of the drop-off and pickup of the child should be maintained.

• **Policies and rules.** Facilities need to have written policies regarding potentially critical children's issues such as age limits, rest-room practices, food, and parental presence on site. Parents must be informed of these policies and subsequently must sign a form indicating that they have received the polices, understand the policies, and will abide by the policies.

• **Background checks.** All staff and independent contractors who work in situations where they may be alone with children must undergo both a criminal background check and a child-abuse clearance, where available.

TABLE 8.3 Recommended NSPI Guidelines on Pool and Whirlpool Chemistry

Water chemical	POOLS			SPAS		
	Min	Ideal	Max	Min	Ideal	Max
Free chlorine (ppm)	1.0	1.0-3.0	3.0	1.0	1.0-5.0	10.0
Combined chlorine (ppm)	None	None	.2	None	None	.2
Bromine (ppm)	2.0	2.0-4.0	4.0	2.0	3.0-5.0	10.0
Ph	7.2	7.4-7.6	7.8	7.2	7.4-7.6	7.8
Total alkalinity (ppm)	60	80-100	180	60	80-100	180
Calcium hardness (ppm)	150	200-400	500-1,000+	150	200-400	500-1,000+
Cyanuric acid (ppm)	10	30-50	150	10	30-50	150

Guidelines for Health/ Fitness Facility Operating Practices

TABLE 8.4 Guidelines for Health/ Fitness Facility Operating Practices

1. Facilities that are staffed during all operating hours should have a manager on duty (MOD) or supervisor on duty (SOD) schedule that specifies which professional staff person has supervisory responsibility for overseeing all operating activities during the hours that the facility is open.

2. Facilities should provide the proper level of qualified staffing in nonactivity areas to assist in serving the members and users and providing support to emergency response situations that might arise.

3. Facilities that are unstaffed during some or all operating hours, and therefore have periods in which no supervision is offered, should provide the appropriate signage to communicate to members and users that the facility is unsupervised, the inherent risks in using the facility, and what steps the members and users should take in the event of a witnessed emergency situation.

4. Facilities should have a written system for cleaning and disinfecting the various areas in the facility.

Health/fitness facility operating practices guideline 1. Facilities that are staffed during all operating hours should have a manager on duty (MOD) or supervisor on duty (SOD) schedule that specifies which professional staff person has supervisory responsibility for overseeing all operating activities during the hours that the facility is open.

In the health and fitness industry, extensive operating hours often are the norm; many facilities are open for members and users 16 to 24 hours a day. With such extensive operating hours, it is important that facilities provide a professional staff person to serve as a manager or supervisor on duty during all operating hours. During that person's designated shift, the MOD serves as the point person for member and user and staff issues and, more important, as the lead person in any emergency response situations that might arise. The MOD needs to be trained and certified in AED and CPR and first aid as well as thoroughly versed in the facility's basic operating procedures.

Health/fitness facility operating practices guideline 2. Facilities should provide the proper level of qualified staffing in nonactivity areas to assist in serving the members and users and providing support to emergency response situations that might arise.

As discussed in chapter 5, some facilities operate with minimal or no staffing, while others function in a fully staffed manner. In addition to the professional fitness staff whose primary responsibilities vary from person to person depending on the assigned role within the facility, facilities should also ensure proper staffing levels for nonphysical activity settings, including the front desk, child care areas, housecleaning, locker rooms, and administrative offices.

Health/fitness facility operating practices guideline 3. Facilities that are unstaffed during some or all operating hours, and therefore have periods in which no supervision is offered, should provide the appropriate signage to communicate to members and users that the facility is unsupervised, the inherent risks in using the facility, and what steps the members and users should take in the event of a witnessed emergency situation.

A number of health/fitness facilities, such as some hotel and corporate fitness centers, do not provide staff to supervise the use of the facility either during a portion of the operating hours or for the entire period of operations. In these instances, a facility should make every effort to provide the appropriate signage that clearly indicates to members and users that they are assuming personal responsibility for engaging in the use of the facility without staff supervision, and that as a result, certain risks (pertaining to the unsupervised environment) exist that they should be prepared to deal with.

Health/fitness facility operating practices guideline 4. Facilities should have a written system for cleaning and disinfecting the various areas in the facility.

According to research sponsored by IHRSA, consumers see facility cleanliness as one of the top five factors that influence their decision to join a particular facility. From a safety perspective, the failure to maintain the proper schedule of cleaning and disinfecting the facilities and equipment can lead to the spread of germs that cause illness. Accordingly, a facility should develop and adhere to a written schedule for cleaning (and disinfecting, where applicable) all areas and relevant equipment in the facility. Furthermore, a facility should maintain written records in that regard. Tables 8.5 to 8.8 provide an overview of the recommended cleaning and disinfecting procedures for fitness areas, locker rooms, pools, gymnasiums, and court facilities.

TABLE 8.5 Recommended Cleaning and Disinfecting Procedures for Fitness and Group Exercise Facilities

Facility area	Cleaning activity	Frequency
Fitness floor	• Remove trash.	Daily
	• Dust all horizontal surfaces.	Daily
	• Clean and disinfect vinyl pads on equipment.	Daily
	• Clean and disinfect equipment frames.	Daily
	• Vacuum carpets and clean stains.	Daily
	• Spot-clean mirrors.	Daily
	• Wash and disinfect hard floor surfaces including all rubber floor surfaces.	Daily
	• Clean HVAC vents.	Daily
	• Clean light fixtures.	Bimonthly
	• Vacuum and clean under all equipment.	Bimonthly
	• Fully clean mirrors and glass surfaces.	Bimonthly
	• Clean carpets.	Bimonthly
	• Clean wall surfaces thoroughly.	Quarterly or annually
		Annually
Group exercise studios	• Remove any trash.	Daily
	• Dry-mop wood floors.	Daily
	• Dust all horizontal surfaces.	Daily
	• Spot-clean mirrors and glass surfaces.	Daily
	• Clean mirrors thoroughly.	Daily
	• Wet-mop wood floors.	Weekly
	• Wash and disinfect rubber floor surfaces.	Daily
	• Clean HVAC ducts.	Bimonthly
	• Clean light fixtures.	Bimonthly
	• Clean audio equipment.	Bimonthly
	• Wash solid walls.	Quarterly to annually
	• Refinish wood floor surfaces.	Annually

TABLE 8.6 Recommended Cleaning and Disinfecting Procedures for Locker Rooms

Daily activities	Bimonthly	Monthly/quarterly/annually
Remove trash and replace liners.	Completely clean mirrors and glass surfaces.	Refill air fresheners or dispensers (monthly).
Refill paper dispensers.	Clean all hard surfaces by scrubbing with machine or similar brush.	Clean grout lines in showers (monthly).
Refill all soap and related dispensers.	Clean and disinfect showers, steam room, sauna, and whirlpool completely.	Clean carpets with bonnet-style cleaner (quarterly).
Dust all surfaces with lint-free cloth.	Clean and dust all HVAC grills and vents.	Extraction-clean carpets (annually).
Spot-clean all mirrors and glass surfaces.	Clean light fixtures.	Wash down all walls (annually).
Spot-clean locker surfaces, doors, and all exposed hardware.	Empty and clean out all dispensers.	
Clean and disinfect sinks, toilets, and urinals.	Empty and clean out all waste receptacles.	
Clean and disinfect sauna, steam room, and whirlpool.	Clean and polish all wood surfaces.	
Vacuum carpets.		
Dust-mop or sweep wood surfaces.		
Wet-mop and disinfect hard floor surfaces.		

TABLE 8.7 Recommended Cleaning and Disinfecting Procedures for Pool Areas

Cleaning activity	Comments
Vacuuming the pool	Pools should be vacuumed daily (using built-in vacuums or automatic vacuum systems). The best time to perform vacuuming is at closing to allow for the appropriate time (5 hours) before allowing members to use the pool.
Cleaning skimmers	This is required only in pool systems that use skimmers. Most modern pools use gutter systems. In busy pools, this should be done on a daily basis.
Cleaning the walls and tile	If the pool is paint, vinyl, or fiberglass, then the cleaning should be done with a nylon brush. This process needs to be done at least monthly and more often in pools with heavy usage. The scum line should be cleaned on a regular basis with a soft brush or cloth.
Backwashing the filter	Backwashing needs to occur on a regular basis. In very busy pools, this can be as often as once a day, but more likely will need to be done weekly. Backwashing normally follows the guidelines of the filter manufacturer and type of filter (sand, diatomaceous earth, or cartridge). A pressure rise of 5 psi is often an indicator that backwashing should occur.

TABLE 8.8 Recommended Cleaning and Disinfecting Procedures for Gymnasiums, Racquet Courts, and Tennis Courts

Facility area	Cleaning activity	Frequency
Gymnasium	• Remove trash.	Daily
	• Dry-mop and dust floors.	Daily
	• Dust all horizontal surfaces.	Daily
	• Spot-clean all glass surfaces.	Daily
	• Clean all glass surfaces thoroughly.	Weekly
	• Tack or wet-mop the wood floors.	Weekly
	• Clean heating, ventilation, and air conditioning (HVAC) filters.	Bimonthly
	• Clean light fixtures.	Bimonthly
	• Refinish wood floors.	Every 2 years
Racquet courts	• Remove trash.	Daily
	• Dry-mop and dust floors.	Daily
	• Dust horizontal surfaces.	Daily
	• Spot-clean walls and glass surfaces.	Daily
	• Remove ball marks.	Daily
	• Tack or damp-mop the floors.	Weekly
	• Thoroughly clean glass surfaces.	Bimonthly
	• Clean HVAC vents.	Bimonthly
	• Clean light fixtures.	Bimonthly
	• Refinish floors (squash should be left unfinished, but sanded).	Annually
Tennis courts	• Remove trash.	Daily
	• Sweep or vacuum hard courts indoors.	Daily
	• Blow outdoor courts to remove debris.	Daily
	• Roll-Dri outdoor hard courts after rain.	Daily
	• Sweep courts and brush lines for clay courts.	Daily
	• Water clay courts.	Daily
	• Scrape hardened material off clay courts.	Weekly
	• Patch low spots on clay courts.	Weekly
	• Jet-broom and sweep hard courts and pressure-wash hard courts.	Weekly
	• Recondition clay courts (add surface material).	Biannually
	• Replace tape on clay courts.	Semiannually to annually
	• Resurface hard courts.	Every 2 to 3 years
	• Resurface clay courts.	Every 3 to 4 years

Signage in Health/ Fitness Facilities

Signage is one of the most important means by which health/fitness facilities communicate with their members and users and the general public. Signage can help convey a variety of messages including hazard warnings, cautionary warnings, instructions on proper use of a piece of equipment, and general facility information. When signage is developed and displayed properly, it allows the desired message to be communicated clearly and in a timely manner. On the other hand, poorly conceived and displayed signage can result in either confusion or a complete failure to communicate the desired message.

Signage can serve many roles in communication in a health/fitness facility (e.g., providing physical directions for members and users, instructing on the safe and effective use of equipment, providing information about facility services, and warning about conditions in the facility that might expose members and users to unwarranted risk). Proper signage plays a critical role in establishing a safer physical activity environment. It should be noted, however, that no label or sign alone can prevent all injuries or ensure that all members and users engage in risk-free practices. In that regard, ASTM International developed and issued F1749-02, titled *Standards for Fitness Equipment and Fitness Facility Safety Signage and Labels,* which sets forth guidelines for signage and labels associated with fitness equipment and fitness facilities that can promote a higher level of safety in a health/fitness facility.

This chapter presents standards and guidelines on signage and its use in a health/fitness facility. Table 9.1 lists the four required standards on signage

in health/fitness facilities, and table 9.3 details the three recommended guidelines on signage in health/fitness facilities.

Standards for Signage in Health/Fitness Facilities

TABLE 9.1 Standards for Signage in Health/Fitness Facilities

1. Facilities must post the appropriate caution, danger, and warning signage in conspicuous locations where existing conditions and situations warrant such signage.

2. Facilities must post the appropriate emergency and safety signage pertaining to fire and related emergency situations, as required by federal, state, and local codes.

3. Facilities must post all required ADA and OSHA signage.

4. All cautionary, danger, and warning signage must have the required signal icon, signal word, signal color, and layout, as specified by the American National Standards Institute (ANSI) and reflected in the ASTM's standards for fitness equipment and fitness facility safety signage and labels.

Health/fitness facility signage standard 1. Facilities must post the appropriate caution, danger, and warning signage in conspicuous locations where existing conditions and situations warrant such signage.

A facility has the responsibility to provide members and users with information about conditions and situations that might expose them to an increased risk of experiencing an injury, health-related problem, or even death. In that regard, the following three types of signage are appropriate:

• **Cautionary signage.** Cautionary signage is designed to alert members and users of the potential risks that exist or the hazardous situations that might arise from using a particular piece of equipment, from circumstances inherent in a given facility area or from their participation in a specific program or service that is offered by the facility. Cautionary signage must provide members and users with both a cautionary statement and a concrete list of actions that are appropriate to avoid the risk indicated in the cautionary statement.

• **Danger signage.** Danger signage is designed to provide members and users with a clear message that indicates that an *imminent* hazardous situation exists, and if that situation is not avoided, serious injury or death may result. Danger signage must provide members and users with a clear statement of the applicable danger and what steps must be taken to avoid that danger or risk.

• **Warning signage.** Warning signage is designed to provide members and users with a clear message indicating that a *potentially* hazardous situation exists and, if it is not avoided, death or serious injury could occur. Warning signage should provide members and users with a clear statement

that warns them of the potential risks that apply to a particular situation and the measures that can be taken to avoid the risks. Table 9.2 offers examples of several situations in which cautionary, danger, and warning signage would be appropriate. In each situation, the basic objective of such signage is specified.

Health/fitness facility signage standard 2. Facilities must post the appropriate emergency and safety signage pertaining to fire and related emergency situations, as required by federal, state, and local codes.

It is imperative that facilities comply with all federal, state, and local laws when it comes to the posting of signage pertaining to fire and related emergency situations. As part of the process, it is recommended that all health/fitness facilities consult with both their local fire department and local city authorities to ensure that they are in full compliance with all fire safety and emergency signage. Factors that such signage must address may include the following:

• **Emergency exit signage.** These signs not only show the location of all emergency exits but also provide directions for how to proceed to these exits.

• **Emergency phone and fire extinguisher location signage.** These signs identify the location of telephones and fire extinguishers and provide instructions for their use.

• **AED and first-aid location signage.** These signs identify the location of all AED units and

TABLE 9.2 Examples of Cautionary and Warning Signage

Sign type	Location	Purpose
Steam room caution	Steam room	Provides people with an indication of the risks involved in using a steam room and the steps they can take to reduce those risks.
Physical activity symptoms and warning	Fitness floor, group exercise studio, racquet court areas	Clarifies the symptoms and warning signs of distress related to exercise and the actions people can take to reduce or eliminate those symptoms.
Warning sign for pools	Aquatic areas and swimming pools	Provides warnings about the danger of certain activities and the need for avoiding certain activities, such as diving in the pool, running in the pool area.
Temperature warning sign	Sauna, steam room, and whirlpool	Warns people of the risk involved in exposure to high temperature and humidity and what actions can be taken to minimize that risk.

first-aid kits and include directions on how to get to these locations.

• **Facility occupancy load and certificate of occupancy.** This signage indicates the maximum number of members and users that are allowed in the facility at any given time, according to local building codes.

Health/fitness facility signage standard 3. Facilities must post all required ADA and OSHA signage.

Both the American with Disabilities Act (ADA) and the Occupational Safety and Health Administration (OSHA) provide explicit regulations regarding the posting of certain signage. For example, OSHA requires that a facility post warning signage for hazardous chemicals and blood-borne pathogens if the member or user may be exposed to either. The ADA expects facilities to provide signage that indicates access points for people with physical challenges as well as certain signage that can be viewed by some individuals who have visual impairments.

Health/fitness facility signage standard 4. All cautionary, danger, and warning signage must have the required signal icon, signal word, signal color, and layout as specified by ANSI and reflected in the ASTM standards for fitness equipment and fitness facility safety signage and labels.

The standards and guidelines from both ANSI and ASTM spell out the specific parameters for appearance required for the design and layout of cautionary, danger, and warning signage, including the color of the sign, the wording to be provided, and the type of icon to be used.

Guidelines for Signage in Health/Fitness Facilities

TABLE 9.3   Guidelines for Signage in Health/Fitness Facilities

1. Facilities should attempt to provide every activity area in the facility with the appropriate safety and warning signage.
2. Facilities should provide message boards, bulletin boards, or similar signage for the

communication and dissemination of relevant information on the facility or of particular interest to the facility's members.

3. Signage should have the proper appearance, readability, and placement in order to clearly display the desired message in a fashion that can easily be understood by the intended audience.

Health/fitness facility signage guideline 1. Facilities should attempt to provide every activity area with the appropriate safety and warning signage.

Every area of a health/fitness facility may have some degree of risk associated with it that varies according to the activities that are conducted in a given space. Accordingly, a facility should provide appropriate signage that alerts its members and users that participation in a particular activity may expose them to certain risks. Table 9.4 presents examples of common safety and warning signage that would be appropriate for given areas within a health/fitness facility.

Health/fitness facility signage guideline 2. Facilities should provide message boards, bulletin boards, or similar signage for the communication and dissemination of relevant information on the facility or of particular interest to the facility's members.

To provide a safer and more enjoyable physical activity experience for members and users, facilities should post pertinent information on appropriate communication sites, such as bulletin boards or message boards that are positioned in highly visible locations throughout the facility. Communications could include updates on facility programs and services, rules and policies of the facility, and even facts about certain staff members and their qualifications. The following examples illustrate the various types of communication pieces that this guideline could address:

• **Facility program calendars and schedules.** Facilities can use these communication tools to share with members and users information about selected activities that will be offered during a specified time period. Examples of these types of tools include group exercise schedules, monthly program calendars, and special-event posters.

• **Facility policies and rules.** Facilities can employ these communication tools to detail to

TABLE 9.4 Examples of Area-Specific Safety and Warning Signage

Activity area	Examples of safety warnings
Fitness floor	• Before using any of the equipment, make sure that a staff person demonstrates the proper use of the equipment. • Exercising may cause conditions such as dizziness, light-headedness, disorientation, exhaustion, or other signs or symptoms that put the exerciser at risk. If you experience any of these warnings, you should cease exercising and contact a member of the staff.
Sauna	• Users should limit themselves to no more than 10 minutes in the sauna to avoid the possibility of heat exhaustion or heatstroke. • Members and users with cardiovascular disease, high blood pressure, or other medical conditions that could be exacerbated by exposure to high temperature should consult a medical professional before entering the sauna.
Swimming pool	• Do not run on the pool deck. • Shower before entering the pool. • Do not dive into the pool.

their members and users the expectations of the facility on fundamental issues, such as operating hours, dress code, age restrictions, and appropriate behavior of users.

• **User comments and suggestions.** Facilities can employ these communication tools as a means whereby members and users can post messages about their experiences in the facility or services relating to the facility on which they would like to provide feedback.

• **Facility staff information.** Facilities can use these communication tools to share information with members and users about key staff and their qualifications. This mechanism can be an especially useful way to provide relevant information about personal trainers and other physical activity instructors.

Health/fitness facility signage guideline 3. Signage should have the proper appearance, readability, and placement in order to clearly display the desired message in a fashion that can easily be understood by the intended audience.

The following points delineate the relevant factors that a facility should consider regarding signage:

• **Appearance.** A sign should use colors and materials that are most likely to communicate the desired message. For instance, it is recommended that the color red be used for danger, orange for warning, and yellow for caution. The type of material used in the sign can also be important. For example, a waterproof material should be used for all signage that is posted in areas exposed to high humidity and water.

• **Readability.** This factor refers to the words, symbols, pictures, and typeface that are used to build the signage. For example, whenever possible, line drawings and illustrations should be used on signage, since they often have universal meaning. Moreover, the use of certain symbols, such as a person falling, can indicate that a condition exists that presents a slip-and-fall danger. Any typeface used on the signage should be bold and large enough so that the reader can easily read the message from a distance.

• **Placement.** This feature refers to the location of signage. Signs should be placed in conspicuous locations that can be easily seen by the user. Signs should be placed at eye level and have sufficient white space or open space around them so that the reader's focus is clearly directed to the signage.

Supplements

Supplement 1

Lighting Guidelines for Selected Outdoor Areas and Activities

Considerations

The following factors must be considered when installing or renovating outdoor lighting systems:

1. In general, overhead lighting is more efficient and economical than low-level lighting.

2. Fixtures should provide an overlapping pattern of light at a height of about 7 ft.

3. Lighting levels should respond to site hazards such as steps, ramps, and steep embankments.

4. Posts and standards should be placed so that they do not create hazards for pedestrians or vehicles.

Notes

1. Because of their effect on light distribution, trees and shrubs at present height and growth potential should be considered in a lighting layout.

2. It is recommended that facilities use manufacturer-provided lighting templates sized for fixture type, wattage, pole height, and layout scale.

3. Facilities should consider color rendition when selecting light source. When possible, colors should be selected under proposed light source.

4. Light pollution to areas other than those to be illuminated should be avoided.

Low-level lighting
1. Heights below eye level
2. Very finite patterns with low wattage capabilities
3. Incandescent, fluorescent, and high-pressure sodium, 5- to 150-W lamps
4. Lowest maintenance requirements, but highly susceptible to vandals

Mall and walkway lighting
1. 10- to 15-ft heights average for multiuse areas; wide variety of fixtures and light patterns
2. Mercury, metal halide, or high-pressure sodium, 70- to 250-W lamps
3. Susceptible to vandals

Special-purpose lighting
1. 20- to 30-ft heights average
2. Recreational, commercial, residential, and industrial
3. Mercury, metal halide, or high-pressure sodium, 200- to 400-W lamps
4. Fixtures maintained by gantry

Parkway and roadway lighting
1. 30- to 50-ft heights average
2. Large recreational, commercial, and industrial areas, and highways
3. Mercury, metal halide, or high-pressure sodium, 400- to 1000-W lamps
4. Fixtures maintained by gantry

High mastlighting
1. 60- to 100-ft heights average
2. Large areas—parking and recreational areas and highway interchanges
3. Metal halide or high-pressure sodium, 1000-W lamps
4. Fixtures must lower for maintainance

Step light
2 ft
Mushroom
Up lights
10-15 ft
Down light
Wide spread down light
Standard globe
Globe with directional refractor
20-30 ft
30-50 ft
60-100 ft

Architectural graphic standards, 8th ed., C.G. Ramsey and H.R. Sleeper. Copyright 1988 by John Wiley & Sons, Inc. Reprinted with permission of John Wiley & Sons, Inc.

Supplement 2
Samples of Signage Used in a Health/Fitness Facility

Sauna Policies

1. The sauna temperature is kept between 170 and 180 °F (77 and 82 °C).
2. Limit yourself to a maximum of 10 minutes.
3. Because of high temperatures, the sauna can be dangerous to your health. We recommend that you consult your physician before you use the sauna. Those who are pregnant and those with medical conditions such as high blood pressure, heart disease, and respiratory problems should avoid exposure to high heat.
4. Allow yourself at least 5 minutes after exercising to cool down before entering.
5. No food or drink is allowed inside.
6. Please shower before entering.

Steam Room Policies

1. The steam room temperature is kept between 100 and 110 °F (38 and 43 °C).
2. Limit yourself to a maximum of 10 minutes.
3. Because of high temperatures and humidity, the steam room can be dangerous to your health. We recommend that you consult your physician before you use the steam room. Those who are pregnant and those with medical conditions such as high blood pressure, heart disease, and respiratory problems should avoid exposure to high heat and humidity.
4. Allow yourself at least 5 minutes after exercising to cool down before entering.
5. No food or drink is allowed inside.
6. Please shower before entering.

Pool Policies

1. The pool temperature is kept between 78 and 84 °F (25 and 29 °C) and is posted daily.
2. Please shower before entering the pool.
3. No diving is allowed.
4. No food or drink is allowed in the pool area.
5. No running or playing is allowed on the pool deck.
6. Individuals with open wounds or sores should not enter the pool.

Racquetball Court Rules

1. Eye guards are required!
2. Black-soled shoes are not allowed on the court.
3. No food or drink is allowed on the court.

Court Numbers Signs

Racquetball Court 1   Squash Court 1
Racquetball Court 2   Squash Court 2
Racquetball Court 3   Squash Court 3

Cardiovascular Area Policies

1. Please limit yourself to 30 minutes on all cardiovascular equipment. During prime times, limit yourself to 20 minutes.
2. Please use the sign-up board when all equipment is taken so people can use the equipment on a first-come, first-served basis.
3. Please wipe off controls, seats, and railings when you are finished with your workout.
4. Please return cardiovascular equipment controls to their start position when your workout is completed.
5. We recommend you see the club's fitness staff before you start a training program.
6. Please warm up before using the equipment and cool down afterward.
7. Please report any injuries to the facility staff.

Resistance Circuit Policies

1. We recommend you see the club's fitness staff before you start a training program.
2. During prime times, please limit yourself to a maximum of two sets per station. You may return after completing the rest of your circuit.
3. Please lower and raise the plates carefully.
4. Please wipe off the pads when you are finished with a piece of equipment.

Free Weight Area Policies

1. We recommend you see the club's fitness staff before you start a training program.
2. Because of the high risk of injury, we recommend you use a spotter when training with free weights.
3. Please replace all dumbbells and plates on the appropriate racks when finished with them.
4. Please remove plates from bars when you are finished with them.

Treadmill Policies

1. Start the treadmill before you step on the belt.
2. Increase the speed and elevation gradually.
3. After completing your workout, gradually reduce the speed to 3 miles per hour and the elevation to 0.
4. Please wipe off the control panel after completing your workout.

Pool Temperature

1. Pool temperature is _____.

   (The blank should be filled in with signage of temperature. Facility operators should create temperature figures from 78 to 86 °F.)

Whirlpool Policies

1. The whirlpool temperature is kept between 102 and 105 °F.
2. Limit yourself to a maximum of 10 minutes.
3. Due to high temperature and humidity, the whirlpool can be dangerous to your health. We recommend that you consult your physician before you use the whirlpool. Those who are pregnant and those with medical conditions such as high blood pressure, heart disease, and respiratory problems should avoid exposure to high heat and humidity.
4. Allow yourself at least 5 minutes after exercising to cool down before entering.
5. No food or drink is allowed in whirlpool.
6. Please shower before entering.

Equipment out of Order

This equipment is out of service. It will be repaired or in service by _____.

Supplement 3

Sample Preventive Maintenance Schedule—
Resistance Equipment

Equipment	Daily	Weekly	Monthly
Selectorized	Clean upholstery with cotton cloth and mild soap solution. Clean frames with cotton cloth and either warm mild detergent or all-purpose liquid cleaner. *Extra* Clean off dumbbell rack with warm mild detergent or all-purpose liquid cleaner.	Lubricate guide rods and linear bearings (wipe clean with dry cotton cloth, then wipe entire length with medium weight oil). Inspect and adjust the following: • Cables • Nuts and bolts • Torn upholstery Apply vinyl upholstery protectant. *Extra* Wipe off dumbbells and barbell plates. Check bolts on bars.	Wash grips in mild soap and water.
Pneumatic	Clean upholstery with cotton cloth and mild soap solution. Wipe off frames with cotton cloth. Release air pressure.	Polish chrome with cotton cloth and automotive chrome polish. Clean seat belts with mild soap. Every two weeks, switch the compressor pump. Apply vinyl upholstery protectant.	Lubricate cylinder rods with dry cotton cloth and lightweight machine oil. Lubricate pivot bearings. Wash rubber handgrips in mild soap and water.

Equipment	Daily	Weekly	Monthly	Biannually
Rower	Clean monorail with nonabrasive pad. Wipe off seat and console with 100% cotton cloth using water and mild detergent (dilute).	Clean and lubricate chain using 100% cotton cloth and lightweight oil. Clean pads with vinyl protectant.	Inspect chain links. Adjust seat rollers. Inspect chain handle. Tighten shock cord.	Replace monitor batteries.
Arm/leg ergometer	Wipe off seat and console with 100% cotton cloth plus water and mild detergent. Rinse.	Clean and lubricate chain with cotton cloth and lightweight machine oil. Clean seat with vinyl protectant.	Inspect bolts.	
Computerized bike	Clean seat and console with 100% cotton cloth and mild soap with water (dilute). Clean housing with same materials.	Clean and lubricate chain with cotton cloth and lightweight machine oil. Clean pedals and lubricate. Wax seat post with auto wax. Clean shroud and seat with vinyl protectant.	Inspect bolts and screws.	
Mechanical stairclimber	Clean console and housing with cotton cloth and water with mild detergent. Wipe and clean pedals and grips with solution from above.	Clean and lubricate all bushings with lightweight machine oil. Clean machine with vinyl protectant.	Inspect housing, belts, and electrical components and repair as needed.	
Treadmill	Clean console and housing with cotton cloth and water with mild detergent solution.	Clean belt with cotton cloth and mild detergent solution. Must run belt at 2 mph while cleaning.	Inspect electrical components and bolts—calibrate if needed (see manual).	
Recumbent bike	Clean housing, console, and seat with cotton cloth and mild soap. Charge battery overnight.	Inspect all bolts and chains and adjust as needed.		

Outline for a Hazard Communication Program

The OSHA Hazard Communication Standard requires you to develop a written hazard communication program. The following is an outline of how to set up your hazard communication.

1. **General company policy.** This must state the organization's intent to comply with OSHA Hazard Communication Standard, Title 29, Code of Federal Regulations 1920.1200. This section should provide an overview of the organization's policy.

2. **List of hazardous chemicals.** This must list chemicals and their locations. It should also mention that lists of chemicals will be posted in the appropriate facility areas.

3. **Material safety data sheets.** This must outline what the chemical compositions and safety hazards of a product are, how they will be posted, and who is in charge.

4. **Labels and other forms of warning.** This section must clearly state that labels and other warnings will be posted on all hazardous materials.

5. **Nonroutine tasks.** This section must describe precautions and training that will be required for nonroutine tasks.

6. **Training.** This section must outline the organization's initial and ongoing training programs that pertain to use and handling of hazardous materials.

7. **Contractor employees.** This section must outline policies for dealing with independent contractors.

8. **Additional information.** This section must direct employees to the appropriate information source for further data.

Based on information from OSHA.

Supplement 6

Sample Organizational Chart

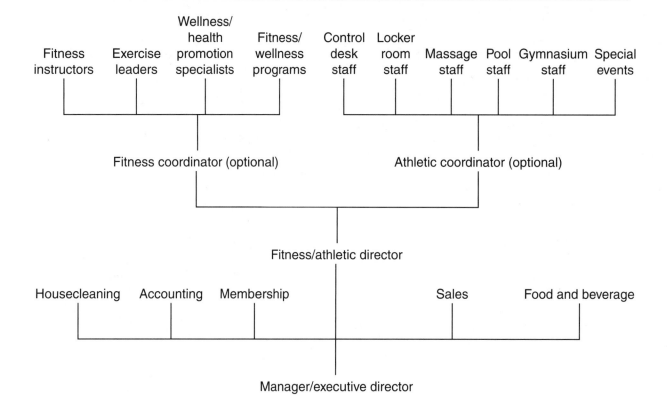

Supplement 7

Supplement 7

Sample Organizational and Staffing Structure

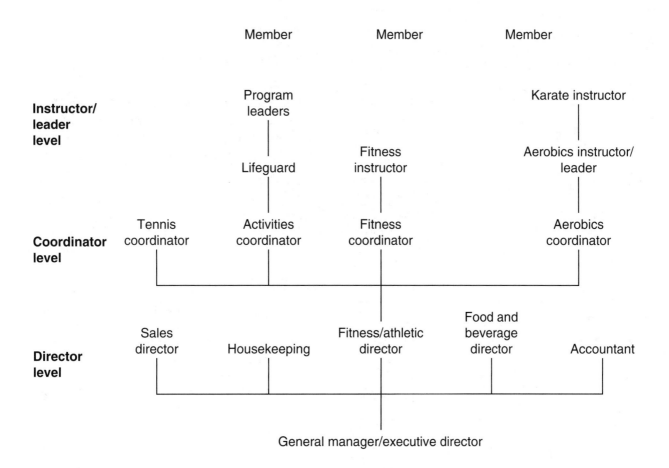

Note. Support staff (e.g., massage therapists, locker room attendants, and control desk staff) will report to someone at the coordinator or director level. Specifically, staff will usually report to someone at the director level.

Supplement 8

Acoustical Guidelines for a Health/Fitness Facility

Owners and managers of health/fitness facilities should incorporate the following noise guidelines into the design and operation of the health/fitness facility.

Area	STC rating	Measured reverberation time
Aerobic studio	45 to 55	.8 to 1.4 s
Control desk	45 to 50	.8 to 1.4 s
Cardiovascular training area	40 to 50	.8 to 1.4 s
Resistance training area	40 to 50	.8 to 1.4 s
Free-weight area	40 to 50	.8 to 1.4 s
Gymnasium	45 to 55	.8 to 1.4 s
Racquetball court	45 to 55	.8 to 1.4 s
Squash court	45 to 55	.8 to 1.4 s
Indoor pool	45 to 55	.8 to 1.4 s
Locker rooms	45 to 50	.8 to 1.4 s
Pro shop area	60 minimum	.8 to 1.4 s
Massage	45 to 55	.8 to 1.4 s
Sports/physical therapy	45 to 55	.8 to 1.4 s
Playroom	50 to 55	.8 to 1.4 s
Offices	50 to 55	.8 to 1.4 s
Storage	40 to 45	.8 to 1.4 s
Indoor tennis courts	45 to 55	.8 to 1.4 s
Laundry area	50 to 60	.8 to 1.4 s
Indoor track area	45 to 55	.8 to 1.4 s

Architectural graphic standards, 8th ed., C.G. Ramsey and H.R. Sleeper. Copyright 1988 by John Wiley & Sons, Inc. Reprinted with permission of John Wiley & Sons, Inc.

RATIONALE

SOUND CONTROL OBJECTIVES

The primary reasons for attempting to control noise within the health/fitness facility involve either increasing the comfort level for facility employees and users or improving communications between occupants of the facility. Although little to no threat of hearing loss from sound abuses exists within the health/fitness facility, high noise levels do cause other problems. Noise can be disruptive and is usually irritating. Noise also hinders an individual's sense of privacy. Perhaps most important, noise can have a negative effect on task performance.

NOISE STANDARDS

Noise is generally measured with sound-pressure meters that record sound in decibels (dB). Minimal acceptable standards for safe noise levels have been established by two federal regulatory agencies—the Occupational Safety and Health Administration (OSHA) and the Environmental Protection Agency (EPA).

NOISE SOLUTIONS

Excessive noise levels can be reduced to acceptable levels by specific actions depending upon the cause of the noise. The two primary sources of unwanted sound—high noise levels and excessive reverberation—can be dampened by adding acoustical absorbents in the affected areas. The degree of insulation of airborne sound provided by a given material is indicated by its sound transmission class (STC) rating. The higher the rating, the better the level of sound absorption. Other methods for diminishing unwanted sound include changing the shape or the layout of an area, using background sound to mask the noise, directly eliminating the cause of the noise (e.g., the stereo system may be too loud), and isolating either the sound or the vibration.

Recommended Maximum Background Noise Criterion Curves for Health and Fitness Facilities

Facility area	NC level	Facility area	NC level
Exercise classroom	35-40	Child care	25-35
Fitness floor	35-40	Racket courts	35-40
Gymnasium	35-40	Pools (indoor)	35-40
Locker rooms	35-40	Offices	30-35
Physical therapy	30-35		

Note. The noise criteria (NC) curves provide a convenient way of defining ambient noise level in terms of octave band sound pressure levels. The NC curves consist of a family of curves relating the spectrum of noise to an environment. Therefore, higher noise levels (decibels) may be allowed at lower frequencies because the ear is less sensitive to noise at lower frequencies.

Architectural graphic standards, 8th ed., C.G. Ramsey and H.R. Sleeper. Copyright 1988 by John Wiley & Sons, Inc. Reprinted with permission of John Wiley & Sons, Inc.

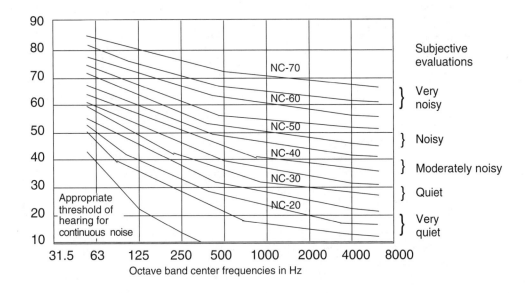

Noise Criteria Sound Pressure Level Table

	Sound pressure level, dB							
NC curve	63 Hz	125 Hz	250 Hz	500 Hz	1000 Hz	2000 Hz	4000 Hz	8000 Hz
NC-70	83	79	75	72	71	70	69	68
NC-65	80	75	71	68	66	64	63	62
NC-60	77	71	67	63	61	59	58	57
NC-55	74	67	62	58	56	54	53	52
NC-50	71	64	58	54	51	49	48	47
NC-45	67	60	54	49	46	44	43	42
NC-40	64	57	50	45	41	39	38	37
NC-35	60	52	45	40	36	34	33	32
NC-30	57	48	41	36	31	29	28	27
NC-25	54	44	37	31	27	24	22	21
NC-20	50	41	33	26	22	19	17	16
NC-15	47	36	29	22	17	14	12	11

Note. For convenience in using noise criteria data, the table lists the sound pressure levels in decibels for the NC curves from the above chart.

Architectural graphic standards, 8th ed., C.G. Ramsey and H.R. Sleeper. Copyright 1988 by John Wiley & Sons, Inc. Reprinted with permission of John Wiley & Sons, Inc.

Supplement 9

Effects of Various Temperatures on Human Performance

Effective temperature (F°)*	Performance effects
90	Upper limit for continued occupancy over any reasonable period of time.
80-90	Expect universal complaints, serious mental and psychomotor performance decrement, and physical fatigue.
80	Maximum for acceptable performance even of limited work; work output reduced as much as 40 to 50%; most people experience nasal dryness.
78	Regular decrement in psychomotor performance; individuals experience difficulty falling asleep and remaining asleep; optimum for bathing or showering.
75	Clothed subjects experience physical fatigue, become lethargic and sleepy, and feel warm; unclothed subjects consider this temperature optimum without some type of protective cover.
72	Preferred for year-round sedentary activity while subjects are wearing light clothing.
70	Midpoint for summer comfort; optimum for demanding visual-motor tasks.
68	Midpoint for winter comfort (heavier clothing) and moderate activity, but slight deterioration in kinesthetic response; people begin to feel cool indoors while performing sedentary activities.
66	Midpoint for winter comfort (very heavy clothing) while subjects are performing heavy work or vigorous physical exercise.
64	Lower limit for acceptable motor coordination; shivering occurs if individuals are not extremely active.
60	Hand and finger dexterity deteriorates, limb stiffness begins to occur, and shivering is positive.
55	Hand dexterity is reduced by 50%, strength is materially decreased, and there is considerable (probably uncontrolled) shivering.
50	Extreme stiffness; strength application accompanied by some pain; lower limit for unprotected exposure for more than a few minutes.

*These temperature effects are based on relatively still air and normal humidity (40 to 60%). Higher temperatures are acceptable if airflow is increased and humidity is lowered (a shift from 1 to 4°); lower temperatures are less acceptable if airflow increases (a shift upward of 1 to 2°).

Supplement 10
General Illumination Guidelines

Task requirements	Light level (FC)	Type of illumination
Small detail; low contrast; prolonged viewing; fast, error-free response	100	Supplementary lighting fixture located near visual task
Small detail, fair contrast, close but short duration work, speed not essential	50-100	Supplementary lighting and/or well-distributed and diffused general lighting
Typical office/desk activity	40-60	General lighting with diffusing fixture directly overhead
Sports (e.g., tennis and basketball) or indoor recreational games (e.g., Ping-Pong and billiards)	30-50	General lighting with sufficient number of fixtures to provide even court or table illumination
Recreational reading and letter writing	25-45	Supplementary lighting, positioned over reading so that page glare does not occur
Typical housekeeping activities	10-25	General lighting
Visibility for moving about, avoiding people and furniture, and negotiating standard stairs	5-10	General and/or supplementary lighting (with care taken not to allow supplementary sources to project in the user's eyes)

Note. These guidelines are only approximations. Foot-candle values are higher than some recommendations, not for seeing, but because these levels provide an additional psychological benefit as well. Levels relate to light levels measured at the primary seeing point (e.g., the desk or table surface, on the floor, or stair tread level). Brightness ratios between the seeing task and the immediate surroundings should not exceed 5:1; between the task and the remote surroundings, 20:1; and between the immediate work area and any other remaining visual environment, 80:1. Natural or white artificial light should be used regardless of the type of illumination (i.e., these levels do not apply to monochromatic light sources).

From W.E. Woodson, 1981, *Human factors design handbook* (New York: McGraw-Hill Companies), 434. Reproduced with permission of The McGraw-Hill Companies.

Supplement 11
DIN Floor Standards

The flooring for a multiuse exercise area should adhere to Deutsches Institut für Normung (DIN) standards. These standards require that a floor meet six criteria:

1. **Shock absorption**—a floor's ability to reduce the impact of contact with the floor surface. The greater the shock absorption, the more protective it is because it reduces impact forces. An aerobics floor, for example, would need more shock absorption than a basketball court.

2. **Standard vertical deformation**—the actual vertical deflection of the floor upon impact. The greater the deformation, the more the floor defects downward. Floors with minimal deformation are not good at absorbing impact forces.

3. **Deflective indentation**—the actual vertical deflection of the floor at a distance 50 cm from the point of impact. The greater the indentation, the more likely impact at one spot will cause deflection at a distant point.

4. **Sliding characteristics**—the surface friction of the finished floor. A floor with poor sliding characteristics would be inappropriate for aerobics or basketball.

5. **Ball reflection (game-action response)**—the response of a ball dropped on the floor compared to a ball dropped on concrete.

6. **Rolling load**—a floor's ability to withstand heavy weight without breaking or sustaining permanent damage.

These DIN criteria are then used to evaluate the effectiveness of a floor. A floor will have one of three functions:

1. **Sports function**—A floor that serves a sports function enhances athletic performance. Surface friction and ball reflection are important here.

2. **Protective function**—A floor that serves a protective function reduces the risk of injury (e.g., from a fall) during activity. Shock absorption is important here.

3. **Material-technical function**—A floor that serves a material-technical function meets the sports and protective functions.

In a health/fitness facility, the gymnasium and multipurpose floors are classified under sports function or material-technical function. The aerobics floor is classified under protective function, with some sports function characteristics.

A floor surface that has a material-technical function should meet the following DIN criteria:

Shock absorption	53% minimum
Standard vertical deformation	2.3 mm minimum
Deflective indentation	15% maximum
Sliding characteristics	0.5 to 0.7 range
Ball deflection	90% minimum
Rolling load	337.6 lb

Supplement 12

Dimensions and Markings for a Basketball Court

Basketball Court and Ball Dimensions

	Court				Basketball		
Type	L (ft)	W (ft)	TP (ft-In)	Type	Max circumference (in.)	Min. circumference (in.)
NBA	94	50	23-9 R	NBA	30	29.5
International	94	50	20-61 R	International	30	29.5
NCAA (men)	94	50	19-9 R	NCAA (men)	30	29.5
WNBA NCAA (women)	94	50	19-9 R	WNBA NCAA (women)	29	28.5
High school (men)	84	50	19-9 R	High school (men)	30	29.5
High school (women)	84	50	19-9 R	High school (women)	29	28.5

L = length, W = width, TP = three point line.

Portable hydraulic goal (plan)

Manual pump or electric control location

14 ft 0 in. playing position

3 ft 6 in.

15 in.
6 in.
18 in. inner diameter
All parts of arc are welded and painted orange

Goal (plan)

5/8 in. diameter steel rod
Breakaway rim with spring
3/8 in. diameter steel rod
12 in.
3/16 in. steel plate
Net 12-mesh, 15 in. to 18 in. long

Goal (elevation)

9 9/16 in. diameter
Basketball

Counterweights (built into frame)
Movable goal ring
11 ft 4 in. folded
Safety locking bar
Hydraulic cylinder
Court line
6 ft 6 in.
9 ft 0 in.
10 ft 0 in.
1 in. high density foam padding
2 in. high density foam padding
6 ft 0 in.
4 ft 0 in.
4 ft 0 in.
3 ft 6 in.

Portable hydraulic goal (elevations)

3 in. white border
1/2 in. tempered glass
2 in. white border
Fully padded
3/8 in. × 2 1/4 in. machine bolts
5 in.
3 in.
3 ft 6 in.
4 ft 0 in.
1 ft 3 in.
5 ft 1 7/8 in.
6 ft 0 in.
9 ft 2 7/8 in. to floor

Backboard (elevation)

2 1/16 in.
6 in.

Section

Note. A basketball court used in high school competition is generally 84 × 50 ft with a 10-ft unobstructed space on all sides (3-ft minimum). A basketball court used in colleges should be 94 ft × 50 ft, with a 10-ft unobstructed space on all sides (3-ft minimum). The color of the lane space marks and neutral zone marks should contrast with the color of the bounding lines. The mid-court marks should be the same color as the bounding lines. All lines should be 2-in. wide (neutral zone excluded). All dimensions are to inside edge of lines except as noted. The backboard should be of any rigid weather-resistant material. The front surface should be flat and painted white unless it is transparent. If the backboard is transparent, it should be marked with a 3-in.-wide white line around the border and an 18-in. × 24-in. target area bounded with a 2-in.-wide white line (DeChiara and Callendar, 1990).

Architectural graphic standards, Version 3.0, C.G. Ramsey. Copyright 2000 by John Wiley & Sons, Inc. Reprinted by permission of John Wiley & Sons, Inc.

Supplement 13

Dimensions and Markings for a Volleyball Court

Court layout

Isometric showing net

Note. The recommended size of a volleyball court is 30 ft × 60 ft with a 10-ft unobstructed area on all sides (6 ft minimum). All measurements for court markings are to be outside of lines except for the centerline. All court markings are to be 2 in. wide, except as noted. Net height at center should be as follows: men 8 ft 0 in., women 7 ft 4 in., high school 7 ft 0 in., elementary school 6 ft 6 in.

From J. DeChiara and J.H. Callendar, 1990, *Time-saver standards for building types*, 3rd ed. (New York: McGraw-Hill Companies), 1212. Reproduced with permission of The McGraw-Hill Companies.

Supplement 14

Dimensions and Markings for a Badminton Court

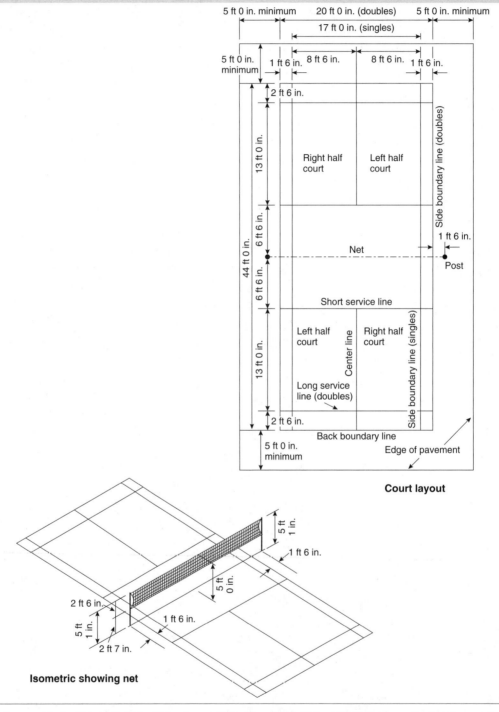

Court layout

Isometric showing net

Note. A singles court for badminton is 17 ft × 44 ft, whereas as doubles court is 20 ft × 44 ft. Both types of badminton courts should have a minimum unobstructed area of 5 ft on all sides. All measurements for court markings are to the outside of the lines except for those involving the center service line, which is equally divided between right and left service courts. All court markings should be 1 1/2 in. wide and preferably white or in color. Minimum distance between sides of parallel courts should be at least 5 ft.

From J. DeChiara and J.H. Callendar, 1990, *Time-saver standards for building types*, 3rd ed. (New York: McGraw-Hill Companies), 1192. Reproduced with permission of The McGraw-Hill Companies.

Supplement 15

Dimensions and Markings for a Racquetball and Handball Court

Note. A standard-size, four-wall racquetball and handball court is 20 ft wide × 40 ft long × 20 ft high. All court markings should be 1 1/2 in. wide and painted white, red, or yellow.

From J. DeChiara and J.H. Callendar, 1990, *Time-saver standards for building types*, 3rd ed. (New York: McGraw-Hill Companies), 1200. Reproduced with permission of The McGraw-Hill Companies.

Supplement 16

Dimensions and Markings
for an International Singles and Doubles Squash Court

Singles squash court

Doubles squash court

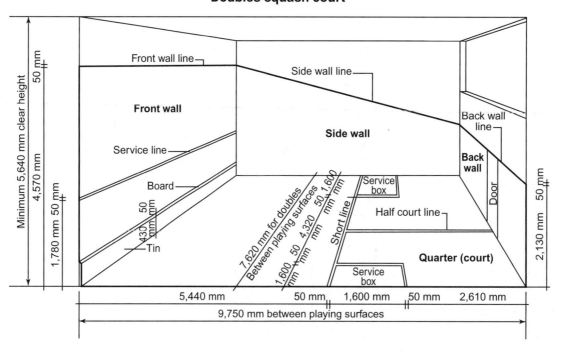

Dimensions for a Singles Squash Court

Length of court between playing surfaces	9,750 mm
Width of court between playing surfaces	6,400 mm
Diagonal	11,665 mm
Height above floor to lower edge of Front Wall Line	4,570 mm
Height above floor to lower edge of Back Wall Line	2,130 mm
Height above floor to lower edge of Service Line on Front Wall	1,780 mm
Height above floor to upper edge of Board	480 mm
Distance to nearest edge of Short Line from Back Wall	4,260 mm
Internal dimensions of Service Boxes	1,600 mm
Width of all lines and the Board	50 mm
Minimum clear height above the floor to the court	5,650 mm

Dimensions for a Doubles Squash Court

Length of court between playing surfaces	9,750 mm
Width of court between playing surfaces	7,620 mm
Diagonal	12,375 mm
Height above floor to lower edge of Front Wall Line	4,570 mm
Height above floor to lower edge of Back Wall Line	2,130 mm
Height above floor to lower edge of Service Line on Front Wall	1,780 mm
Height above floor to upper edge of Board	480 mm
Distance to nearest edge of Short Line from Back Wall	4,260 mm
Internal dimensions of Service Boxes	1,600 mm
Width of all lines and the Board	50 mm
Minimum clear height above the floor to the court	5,640 mm

Notes

1. The Side Wall Line is angled between the Front Wall Line and the Back Wall Line.

2. The Service Box is a square formed by the Short Line, the Side Wall, and two other lines marked on the floor.

3. The length, width, and diagonal of the court are measured at a height of 1,000 mm above the floor.

4. It is recommended that the Front Wall Line, Side Wall Line, Back Wall Line, and Board are shaped so as to deflect any ball that strikes them.

5. The Board shall not project from the Front Wall by more than 45 mm.

6. It is recommended that the door to the court is in the center of the Back Wall.

7. The general configuration of a Squash Court, its dimensions, and its markings are illustrated on the above diagram.

Construction

A Squash Court may be constructed from a number of materials providing they have suitable ball rebound characteristics and are safe for play; however, the WSF publishes a Squash Court Specification, which contains recommended standards. The standards must be met for competitive play as required by the appropriate National Governing Body of Squash.

Court constructors are advised that where events involve professional players the height above floor to the top of the board may be reduced from 480mm to 430mm. If you are considering holding a professional tournament please check with the World Squash Federation office for the latest guidelines.

Supplement 17

Dimensions and Markings for a Tennis Court

Court layout

Isometric showing net

Note. The playing area of a tennis court is 36 ft × 78 ft with at least 12 ft clearance on both sides or between a series of adjacent courts and 21 ft clearance on each end. All measurements for court markings are to the outside of lines except for those involving the center service line, which is equally divided between the right and left service courts. All court markings should be 2 in. wide. Fence enclosure, if provided, should be 10 ft high, 11-gauge, 1-3/4 in. mesh chain link.

From J. DeChiara and J.H. Callendar, 1990, *Time-saver standards for building types*, 3rd ed. (New York: McGraw-Hill Companies), 1210. Reproduced with permission of The McGraw-Hill Companies.

Supplement 18

Dimensions and Markings for a Platform Tennis Court

Court layout

Isometric showing fence (typical wood construction)

Note. The playing area of a platform tennis court is 20 ft × 44 ft, with an 8-ft space on each end and a 5-ft space on each side. All measurements for court markings are to be outside of lines except for those involving the center service line, which is equally divided between the right and left service court. All court markings should be 2 in. wide. Fencing is required—12 ft high with 16-gauge hexagonal, galvanized 1-in. flat wire mesh fabric. The net should be 3 ft 1 in. high at posts and 2 ft 10 in. at the center court.

From J. DeChiara and J.H. Callendar, 1990, *Time-saver standards for building types*, 3rd ed. (New York: McGraw-Hill Companies), 1208. Reproduced with permission of The McGraw-Hill Companies.

Supplement 19

Dimensions and Markings for a Paddle Tennis Court

Court layout

Isometric showing net

Note. The playing area of a paddle tennis court is 20 ft × 50 ft, plus a 15-ft (minimum) space on each side and a 10-ft (minimum) space on each side or between an adjacent court. All measurements for court markings are to the outside of lines except for those involving the center service line, which is equally divided between the right and left service court. All court markings should be 1 1/2 in. wide. Fence enclosure, if provided, should be 1 1/2 in. mesh, 11-gauge chain link.

From J. DeChiara and J.H. Callendar, 1990, *Time-saver standards for building types*, 3rd ed. (New York: McGraw-Hill Companies), 1209. Reproduced with permission of The McGraw-Hill Companies.

Supplement 20

Illumination Requirements[1]
for Different Competitive Levels of Indoor Tennis Play

	ILLUMINATION LEVEL[2] FOR CLASS OF PLAY			
	I	II	III	IV
Description of the facility	Professional, international, national, and college	College, regional, municipal, club, and residential	Club, high school, instructional, parks, and residential	Parks and recreational
Average maintained horizontal illumination[3] within PPA (FC)	125	75	60	50
Minimum maintained horizontal illumination within PPA (FC)	100	60	50	40
Maximum uniformity ration within primary playing area (FC) — CV	.10 or less	.10 or less	.13 or less	.17 or less
Maximum uniformity ration within primary playing area (FC) — E_{max}/E_{min}	1.5:1 or less	1.5:1 or less	1.7:1 or less	2.0:1 or less

[1]Coordinated with the United States Tennis Association.
[2]Illuminance readings should be taken at a 1-meter (3-foot) elevation.
[3]Maintained minimum illuminance is the lowest maintained light level at any measurement or calculation point.

Material derived from the IESNA *Recommended Practice for Sports and Recreational Area Lighting,* with permission from IESNA.

Supplement 21

Basic Comparative Advantages and Disadvantages of the Three Primary Sources of Lighting for Outdoor Courts

Source	Advantages	Disadvantages
High-intensity discharge	Long lamp life High efficiency	Fairly large and heavy Requires a warm-up time of 3 to 7 min to achieve maximum light output
Incandescent (e.g., quartz, iodine, tungsten, halogen)	Low initial cost High color acceptability Excellent light control Relatively small in size and weight Instantaneous starting Capability of using coin- or token-operated meters	Short lamp light High maintenance and operating costs due to low efficacy
Fluorescent	Daylight color Immediate relight time Lower mounting height for easy maintenance High efficiency	Undesirable glare Relatively low brightness Requires a ballast to operate

Supplement 22

Illumination Requirements[1]
for Different Competitive Levels of Outdoor Tennis Play

		ILLUMINATION LEVEL[2] FOR CLASS OF PLAY			
		I	II	III	IV
Description of the facility		Professional, international, national, and college	College, regional, municipal, club, and residential	Club, high school, instructional, parks, and residential	Parks and recreational
Average maintained horizontal illumination[3] within PPA (FC)		125	75	50	30
Minimum maintained horizontal illumination within PPA (FC)		100	60	40	20
Maximum uniformity ration within primary playing area (FC)	CV	.10 or less	.13 or less	.17 or less	.21 or less
	E_{max}/E_{min}	1.5:1 or less	1.7:1 or less	2.0:1 or less	2.0:5 or less

[1]Coordinated with the United States Tennis Association.
[2]Illuminance readings should be taken at a 1-meter (3-foot) elevation.
[3]Maintained minimum illuminance is the lowest maintained light level at any measurement or calculation point.

Material derived from the IESNA *Recommended Practice for Sports and Recreational Area Lighting,* with permission from IESNA.

Supplement 23

Safety Checklist for Pool Areas

Inspection by _____ Date _____

Staff members are expected to report safety factors needing attention on a daily basis so that users are not exposed to unnecessary risks. Managers will make a complete written assessment of the condition of the facility on a regular basis.

Yes   No

Lifesaving equipment

___ ___ Lifeguard stations are strategically located on decks near edge of pool.

___ ___ Shepherd's crooks, spine boards, reaching poles, and ring buoys are consistently placed in a conspicuous and appropriate location.

Pool and deck areas

___ ___ All deck areas are in safe condition.

___ ___ The decks are free of standing water.

___ ___ The sunbathing area is free of any dangerous conditions.

___ ___ The fence that encloses the pool area is in safe condition.

___ ___ All rules and regulations are posted in high-traffic areas such as entrances to the locker rooms. Special rules and regulations such as those on using the diving boards are posted in appropriate locations.

___ ___ All diving boards and stands are properly anchored and in good condition.

___ ___ Water clarity is such that the main drain is clearly visible on the bottom of the pool from the pool deck.

___ ___ All pool markings (depth/warning signs) are clearly visible.

___ ___ All matting on guard platforms is fastened securely and is in safe condition.

___ ___ Diving board steps and railings are fastened securely and are in safe condition.

___ ___ All chairs, cots, and lounges are in safe condition.

Guard room

___ ___ A copy of the procedures for emergencies is posted next to the telephone.

___ ___ Emergency phone numbers are also posted next to the telephone.

___ ___ A first-aid kit with all the necessary emergency first-aid essentials is consistently stored in a conspicuous location.

Filter and chlorinator rooms

___ ___ All motor shafts and filter and soda ash pumps are covered with metal guards.

___ ___ Fire extinguishers (Type B or C), filled and sealed and with current date tags, are kept in strategic locations.

___ ___ All chemicals are stored according to the manufacturer's storage instructions.

___ ___ Antichlorine gas mask is in operative condition. Mask is located immediately outside the entrance to the chlorine room. Canister element has a current, valid date.

___ ___ All gas chlorine tanks are fastened to the wall.

___ ___ Covers to powdered chemicals are fastened tightly and containers are neatly stored.

Locker rooms

___ ___ All floors are kept as dry as possible and are inspected for possible slippery or unsafe conditions.

___ ___ Basket/locker racks are secured to the wall or floor base and are in safe condition.

___ ___ Baskets are in place in the racks.

___ ___ All benches are secured to the wall. Bench tops are finished and free of any rough, splintered edges.

___ ___ All bather signs for pool users are displayed on the walls at appropriate heights.

___ ___ All shower-room plumbing is securely fastened to the walls, and is in safe and operable condition.

___ ___ All walls and ceilings are in safe condition.

___ ___ All lamps light when the switches are turned on.

___

Note. Completed checklists are valuable for several reasons. They are important tools for eliminating the avoidable injury. They also are tangible evidence that a pool manager has concern for the health and safety of pool patrons. In litigation alleging that an unsafe condition on the premises was the cause of the plaintiff's injuries, a completed checklist, signed and dated, could be invaluable. This checklist is incomplete. The items included are examples of safety checks that should be made. To be complete, the checklist should be tailored to a particular facility. Records of safety inspections should be kept indefinitely.

Supplement 24
Dimensions and Markings for a 25-Yard Pool

Note. Twenty-five yards is the minimum length pool for American records. In reality, the pool should be 76 ft 1-1/2 in. long to allow for electronic timing panels to be placed at one end. Twenty-five yard pools should have a minimum of six lanes (45 ft wide), while 10 lanes (83 ft wide) are recommended.

Architectural graphic standards, student edition, 7th ed., R. T. Packard and S.A. Kliment. Copyright 1997 by John Wiley & Sons, Inc. Reprinted by permission of John Wiley & Sons, Inc.

Supplement 25

Dimensions and Markings for a 50-Meter Pool

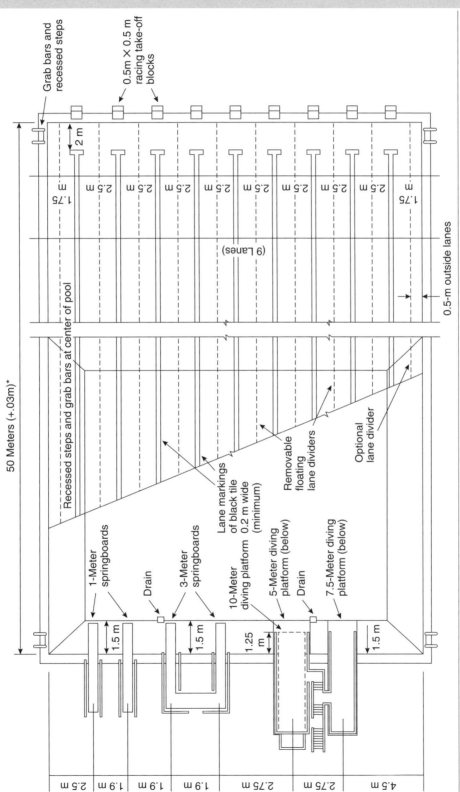

Grab bars and recessed steps

0.5m × 0.5 m racing take-off blocks

2 m

1.75 m | 2.5 m | 2.5 m | 2.5 m | 2.5 m | 2.5 m | 2.5 m | 2.5 m | 2.5 m | 1.75 m

(9 Lanes)

0.5-m outside lanes

Recessed steps and grab bars at center of pool

50 Meters (+.03m)*

Lane markings of black tile 0.2 m wide (minimum)

Removable floating lane dividers

Optional lane divider

1-Meter springboards

Drain

3-Meter springboards

10-Meter diving platform

5-Meter diving platform (below)

Drain

7.5-Meter diving platform (below)

1.5 m

1.5 m

1.25 m

1.5 m

2.5 m | 1.9 m | 1.9 m | 1.9 m | 2.75 m | 2.75 m | 4.5 m

Note. The pool should actually be 50.03 m, allowing an extra 0.03 m to compensate for possible future structural defects electrical timing devices, or tile facing. Fifty meters is the minimum pool length for world records.

Architectural graphic standards, student edition, 7th ed., R.T. Packard and S.A. Kliment. Copyright 1997 by John Wiley & Sons, Inc. Reprinted by permission of John Wiley & Sons, Inc.

Supplement 26

Recommended Diving Pool and Platform Dimensions for Competitive Swimming Programs

Board type	Board size			Distances*			
	Length	Width	Height above water level	A — From edge of pool to end of board	B — From center of board to side of pool	C — From center of board to center of board	D — From end of board to wall ahead
1-meter springboard	16 ft	20 in.	3 ft 3 in.	A-1 7 ft 5 ft	B-1 10 ft 8 ft	C-1 8 ft 6 ft	D-1 28 ft 25 ft
3-meter springboard	16 ft	20 in.	9 ft 11 in.	A-3 7 ft 5 ft	B-3 15 ft 12 ft	C-3 10 ft 8 ft	D-3 33 ft 30 ft
5-meter platform	18 ft	7 ft	16 ft 5 in.	A-5 7 ft 5 ft	B-5 15 ft 12 ft	C-5 10 ft 8 ft	D-5 43 ft 35 ft
10-meter platform	20 ft 20 ft	8 ft 10 ft	32 ft 10 in.	A-10 8 ft 5 ft	B-10 20 ft 15 ft	C-10 10 ft 8 ft	D-10 52 ft 45 ft

Note. The dimensions in the accompanying table are based upon recommended Olympic requirements. Minimum requirements can be satisfied with a pool 35 ft × 45 ft but a somewhat larger size, for example, 60 ft × 60 ft, is recommended. A water-curling arrangement should be provided so that the diver can see exactly where the surface of the water is. If outdoors, the boards should be oriented so that the sun is not in the diver's eyes. Underwater observation parts are desirable. Diving does not require a very large pool, but it must be deep, with at least a 14-ft depth below a 10-m platform.

*Preferred dimensions appear in the left-hand side of a column, while the minimum safe dimensions are listed in the right-hand side of a column.

From J. DeChiara and J.H. Callendar, 1990, *Time-saver standards for building types*, 3rd ed. (New York: McGraw-Hill Companies), 1269. Reproduced with permission of The McGraw-Hill Companies.

Supplement 27

Advantages and Disadvantages of Selected Types of Pool Overflow Systems

Type	Advantages	Disadvantages
Fully recessed gutter	None	Old-fashioned system Most expensive to build Difficult to clean Contrary to efficient pool operation
Semirecessed gutter	Provides visible pool edge for competition Cuts down surface roughness when gutters are flooded Water surface closer to deck than in fully recessed gutter	Water level 5 or 6 inches below deck; difficult for users to climb out of pool Some cleaning difficulty Requires pipe tunnel for access Narrow edge of gutter lip provides precarious footing for diving off edge
Roll-out gutter	Comfortable pool use and egress Ideal for teaching and recreation Gives beginner swimmers feeling of security by allowing wide visibility Easy cleaning Low construction costs	Decks may flood if adequate number of drains not provided Pool edge not visible for competition; temporary turning boards can be used Requires pipe tunnel for access
Deck-level or rimflow system	Trench serves as integral surge tank Minimum construction costs No pipe tunnel needed Comfortable pool use and egress Ideal for teaching and recreation Gives beginner swimmers feeling of security Easy cleaning	Deck can flood if not properly pitched Pool edge not visible for competition; temporary turning boards can be used Care needed in choosing cleaning materials for deck because some deck water enters pool recirculation system Bottom inlets in rimflow system inaccessible for servicing
Surface skimmers	No surge tank required Suitable for very small pools only	Continuing expense and nuisance of maintaining the moveable weirs Turbulence not eliminated in large pools
Prefabricated stainless steel recessed gutter	Pipe tunnel not required Large diameter return pipe is substituted by the manufacturer for a surge tank	Skimmer weirs need manual adjustments several times a day Waterline inlets disturb swimmers in end lanes Exposed rings for lane and lifelines

Supplement 28

Agencies That Offer Construction Standards for Aquatic Facilities and Associations That Serve the Field of Aquatics

American National Standards Institute
1430 Broadway
New York, NY 10018

American Public Health Association
17th and D St., NW
Washington, DC 20006

Council for National Cooperation in Aquatics
(CNCA)
901 W. New York St.
Indianapolis, IN 46202

FINA
208-3540 West 41st Ave.
Vancouver, BC
Canada V6N E36

National Collegiate Athletic Association
(NCAA)
P.O. Box 1906
Shawnee Mission, KS 66201

National Sanitation Foundation
P.O. Box 1468
Ann Arbor, MI 48106

National Spas and Pool Institute (NSPI)
2111 Eisenhower Ave.
Alexandria, VA 22314

U.S. Diving
901 W. New York St.
Indianapolis, IN 46202

U.S. Swimming and U.S. Synchronized Swimming
1750 E. Boulder St.
Colorado Springs, CO 80909

Supplement 29

Dimensions and Markings for a Softball Field for 12-Inch Softball

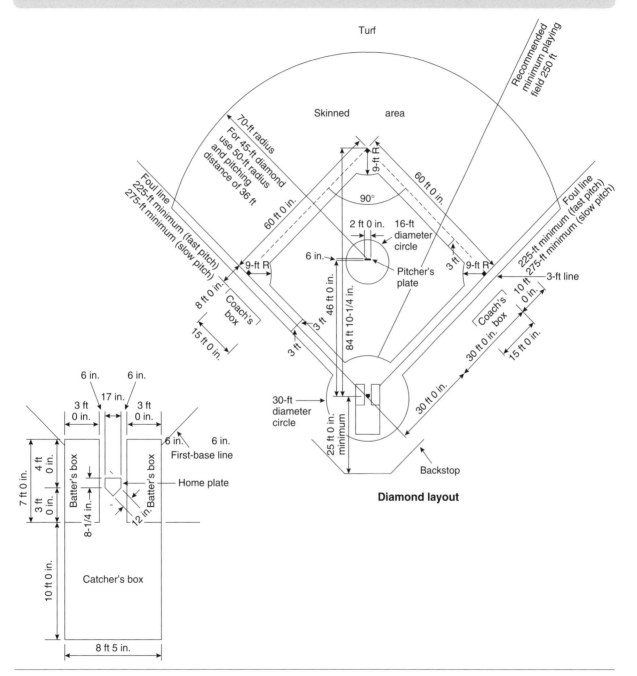

Diamond layout

Note. The recommended baselines are 60 ft for adults and 45 ft for juniors. Distances from home plate to the mound are 46 ft for men, 50 ft for women, and 35 ft for juniors. Juniors should use 45 ft between bases. A field for adult fast-pitch softball should have a 225-ft radius from home plate between the lines. A slow-pitch field has a 275-ft radius and a 250-ft radius for men and women, respectively. The backstop should be located at least 25 ft behind home plate. The foul lines; catcher's, batter's, and coach's boxes; and 3-ft lines should be marked with 2- to 3-in. chalk lines.

From J. DeChiara and J.H. Callendar, 1990, *Time-saver standards for building types*, 3rd ed. (New York: McGraw-Hill Companies), 1227. Reproduced with permission of The McGraw-Hill Companies.

Supplement 30

Dimensions and Markings for a Soccer Field

Playing field layout

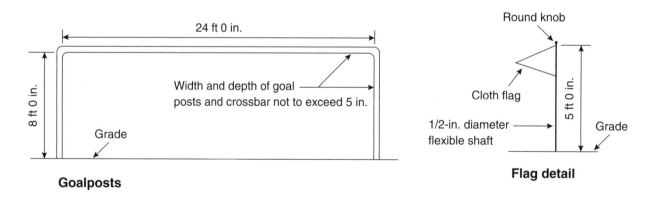

Goalposts

Flag detail

Note. A full-size soccer field is 195 to 225 ft wide by 330 to 360 ft long, with a minimum unobstructed area of 10 ft on all sides. A soccer field for juniors (and in some instances, women) is usually proportionally smaller. Goalposts should be pressure treated with a paintable, oil-borne preservative and painted above ground with three coats of white lead and oil. The goalposts and crossbar should present a flat surface to the playing field, not less than 4 in. or more than 5 in. in width. Nets should be attached to the posts, crossbar, and ground behind the goal. The top of the net must extend backward 2 ft level with the crossbar. All dimensions are to the inside edge of lines. All lines should be 2 in. wide and marked with a white, nontoxic material that is not injurious to the eyes or skin.

From J. DeChiara and J.H. Callendar, 1990, *Time-saver standards for building types*, 3rd ed. (New York: McGraw-Hill Companies), 1225. Reproduced with permission of The McGraw-Hill Companies.

Supplement 31

Playground Equipment Dimensions

Adjacent slides, 7 ft 6 in.

2 ft 0 in.

Swings

Swings	H(ft)	Safety zone A(ft)	Safety zone B(ft)
2	8	24	27
	10	28	27
	12	32	27
3	8	24	30
	10	28	30
	12	32	30
4	8	24	40
	10	28	40
	12	32	40
6	8	24	46
	10	28	46
	12	32	46
8	8	24	57
	10	28	57
	12	32	57
9	8	24	61
	10	28	61
	12	32	61

Slides

H	L	Safety zone A	Safety zone B
4	8	26	24
5	10	26	28
6	12	26	32
8	16	26	36

Horizontal ladder

H (ft, in.)	L (ft, in.)	Safety zone A (ft)	Safety zone B (ft)
6, 6	12, 6	14	25
7, 6	16, 0	14	30

10 ft to 14 ft

General planning information

Equipment	Area (Sq ft)	Capacity (Number of Children)
Slide	450	4–6
Low swing	150	1
High swing	250	1
Horizontal ladder	375	6–8
Seesaw	100	2
Junior climbing gym	180	8–10
General climbing gym	500	15-20

Seesaws

Boards	1	2	3	4	6
L	3	6	9	12	18
A	20	20	20	20	20
B	5	10	15	20	25

Combination units*

Enclosure limits

A = W + 12 ft 0 in.
B = L + 6 ft 0 in.

*Types and number of units are variable

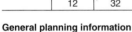

Limits:
A = 8 ft 0 in.
B = L + 6 ft 0 in. heights adjustable
Horizontal bars

Limits:
general 18 ft × 18 ft
junior: 10 ft × 12 ft

General:
8 ft 1-1/2 in.

Junior:
4 ft 6 in.

General:
6 ft 1-1/2 in.
Junior:
6 ft 0 in.

General unit: 9 ft 0 in.
Junior unit: 6 ft 4 in.

N.Y.C. Housing Authority standard climbing gym

18ft – 22ft

10 ft 0 in.

10 ft diameter is considered standard
Other diameters: 6 ft and 8 ft

Spin around

Supplement 32
Outdoor Running Track Lane-Marking Guidelines

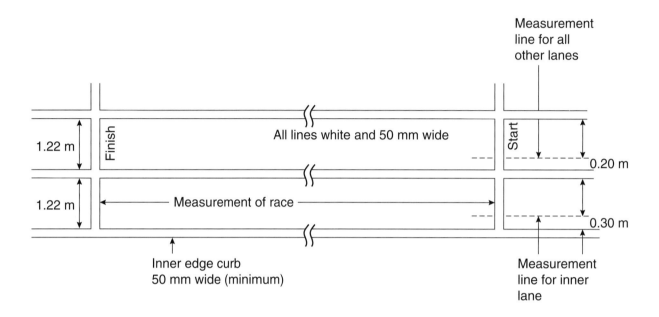

Note. Each lane should be clearly marked and should be a minimum of 1.22 m and a maximum of 1.25 m wide. Each line should be marked by lines 50 mm in width. The inside line of the inside lane should be measured from 0.30 m outward from the inner board of the track. All other lanes should be measured 0.20 m from the outer edge of the preceding line. Tracks used for competition should have a minimum of six lanes; if possible, eight lanes.

Architectural graphic standards, student edition, 7th ed., C.G. Ramsey. Copyright 1997 by John Wiley & Sons, Inc. Reprinted by permission of John Wiley & Sons, Inc.

Supplement 33

Dimensions and Markings for a 440-Yard Running Track

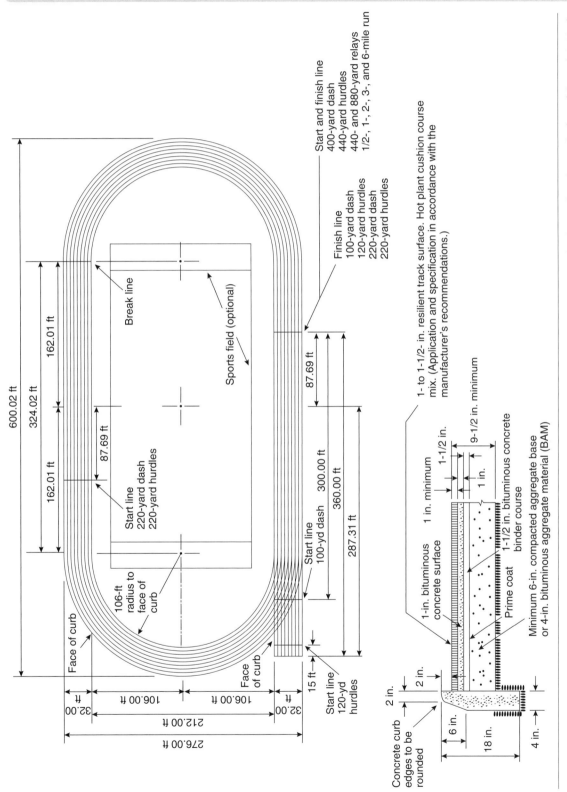

Note. With eight 4-ft-wide lanes, the overall length of a 1/4-mi running track is 600.02 ft. The overall width is 276 ft. The inside radius to the face of the curb is 106 ft. The width of the track is 32 ft. The field-space area inside the track could be marked and used for field sports (e.g., soccer or touch football).

From J. DeChiara and J.H. Callendar, 1990, *Time-saver standards for building types*, 3rd ed. (New York: McGraw-Hill Companies), 1231. Reproduced with permission of The McGraw-Hill Companies.

Supplement 34
Components of a First-Aid Kit

At a minimum, a first-aid kit should contain the following:

- Assorted basic plastic adhesive bandages, various sizes
- 3" × 3" sterile gauze pads (wound dressing)
- 4" × 4" sterile gauze pads (wound dressing)
- 5" × 9" sterile dressing (major wound dressing)
- 3" cohesive bandage (dressing cover)
- Adhesive tape, 2" width (secure dressings, strapping)
- Paper tape, 1" width
- Medical-grade, nonlatex, disposable gloves
- CPR breathing barrier, such as a pocket facemask
- Conforming roller gauze bandage
- Triangular bandages (slings, support, padding)
- Germicidal hand wipes or waterless alcohol-based hand sanitizer
- Antiseptic wipes
- If ice is not immediately available, instant cold packs
- Scissors (first-aid type)
- Tweezers
- Sterile eye pads (emergency eye cover)
- Sterile irrigation solution (wound cleaning, eye wash)
- Emergency blanket
- Current first-aid guide

Supplement 35

AED Prearrival Checklist: Preparing Your Team for AEDs

The following checklist is a quick reference that will help you prepare your employees and members for the arrival of your AED (automated external defibrillator).

____ Review this checklist and the accompanying materials in your AED binder.

____ Pay particular attention to the following sections of this binder, as they will help you the most in preparing for this important program:

- AED policy
- Emergency procedure template
- American Heart Association materials
- AED information
- Support services listing

____ Set up a meeting with your department heads to review the relevant information and discuss your club's strategy (provide handouts of the important information). **During this meeting identify one department head or employee partner to become your AED program coordinator. In addition, discuss how you want to communicate to your members.**

____ Identify the employees who will be part of the initial CPR/AED training. We suggest that these be employees who serve as department heads or employees who cover all of the club's operating hours.

____ Have your AED coordinator set up an AED binder that can be used to store all of the important information, such as the physician's prescription, list of certified employees, weekly operating checklist, AED manual, and club's emergency plan.

____ Have your AED coordinator work with the AED trainer (see the list in your binder) and the AED provider to make sure dates are set up for the training and installation of the program (a calendar of the scheduled training and installation dates will be provided).

____ Establish your club's specific emergency policies so this can be shared with the entire team at a later date.

____ Please note that the AED provider will provide both your physician prescription (standing order) and registration of your AED with the state and local EMS authorities.

____ Arrange a meeting with your entire employee team and share with them the core information about the program and how the club will be implementing the program. Share with them the policies, club emergency plan, proposed member communications, and a list of those who will be receiving training.

____ Arrange to give a presentation to both your board and your committees. Share with them the key information about the program. Discuss with them how to communicate about the AED program to the entire membership.

____ Set up a time line for ongoing training and rehearsal of your program and make it a part of your ongoing operations.

____ Have your AED coordinator make the final arrangements for the training and installation of the club's AED.

Supplement 36
AED Postarrival Checklist:
Creating a Safe Member Environment

This checklist is intended as a quick reference to help you ensure that your team is ready to operate a safe PAD (public access defibrillation) in the club.

____ Make sure that each employee who participates in the AHA Heartsaver AED training receives the proper verification of certification from the AED manager (AHA trainer). Make sure a copy of the certification is placed in the employee's file. You might also consider having a place where you post the names of employees certified in the use and administration of an AED. **Note: You should also place the name of all certified staff in the Web-based AED manager program, which will allow you to monitor the club's staff readiness.**

____ Make sure that the AED provider provides your team and your AED coordinator with complete training in the AED functioning before the AED is actually placed in the club. In addition, make sure the AED coordinator has received complete training in the use of the AED manager program. The AED provider will also indicate the best location for your AED.

____ Have your AED coordinator use the AED manager program on a weekly basis. The following are the requirements for use of this program: enter on a weekly or monthly basis the state of readiness of the AED (you will be shown how to do this) and enter the names of all staff who are certified in CPR and AED use and related information that needs to be entered.

____ The AED manager program will e-mail you when it is time for retraining and recertifying staff, when it is time to replace a battery or pad, and when they notice you are not monitoring the equipment as specified. They will also forward automatically at no cost any replacement battery or pads when the system indicates they need to be replaced.

____ Set up an ongoing rehearsal schedule for dealing with emergencies and in particular the administration of the AED. **It is recommended that you hold rehearsals at least once every 6 months. We are providing as part of this program an AED training regimen that allows you to simulate the actual application of the AED. Take advantage of it and rehearse often.**

____ The AED provider is scheduled to make an annual site inspection to test the AED. Make sure that this happens, as it is backup for your weekly and monthly check-ups.

____ If the event you have to use the AED, make sure to follow the guidelines provided in both this binder and in your training as it applies to recording of the event and communicating said event to your designated medical director. You will also need to coordinate the downloading of all event information to the appropriate medical authority. **Please note that the records of any event can be shared only with the medical director overseeing the AED program unless the member or guest indicates in writing otherwise (HIPAA [health insurance portability and accountability act]).**

____ **In the event you have to use the AED, make sure that you immediately complete an incident report and maintain it on file at the club. In addition, complete the event data sheet on the AED manager program, as this will allow immediate communication with AED managers.**

____ Always keep at least two sets of the following on site with your AED: pads, batteries, and rescue kits. When you use one, immediately replace it.

Supplement 37

Public Access Defibrillation Program: Ongoing Readiness Checklist

Monthly Activities the Club Must Perform

- Make sure your club has a designated AED coordinator who is responsible for the program at the club level and is a registered user of the AED manager system.

- The AED coordinator must check the AED readiness status at least once a month by going to the AED and checking the status indicator for a green check. A red X means it is not working.

- The AED coordinator must access the AED manager Web site for the club at a minimum of once a month. Upon accessing the Web site, the AED coordinator must do the following:

  ___ Indicate that the AED unit was checked and indicate the status as either working or not (green check indicates it is working, red X means it is not working).

  ___ Update the section for certified AED employees if any certified employee has left the club or if a newly certified employee partner is added.

  ___ Update the AED location section if for some reason the AED has been moved or another AED has been added to the club.

- Review your e-mail for any messages that might be forwarded by the AED manager. The AED manager will e-mail notices when it is time to replace pads or batteries as well as when they notice your AED unit has not been checked.

- When a new employee is hired, make sure that person gets an AED certification within 90 days.

- Have an AED certified employee on duty at the club during all operating hours.

Ongoing Activities (As Needed, Semiannual, and Annual) the Club Must Perform

- Conduct practice AED and emergency drills at least twice a year with your staff.

- Provide refresher AED training at least once a quarter using the practice AED unit and dummy that was provided at the time of your AED installation.

- Maintain the number of AED certified employees on staff at a minimum of 10; when the opportunity arises, make every effort to increase that number.

- Have an annual certification class conducted exclusively by the AED manager. This will ensure that you always have enough certified employees in the club, that a third party has verified the clinical integrity/readiness of your AED program, and that all on-site information is updated in the AED Manager system.

- In the event your club has an incident that requires the use of the AED, make sure that, after following the proper emergency procedures, you contact the AED manager and complete the incident follow-up procedures within 24 hours.

- Meet with your department heads and other key supervisors at least twice annually to review the various requirements of the program using the AED program information you received at the time of implementation.

- Replace batteries and pads as directed by the AED manager (every two years) or after an incident.

- Maintain an extra battery and set of pads at the club at all times.

Forms

This appendix contains sample forms for use in health and fitness facilities. The law varies from state to state—no form should be adopted or used by any program without individualized legal advice.

1. Physical Activity Readiness Questionnaire (PAR-Q)
2. Health History Questionnaire
3. Guest Health History Questionnaire
4. Physician's Statement and Clearance Form
5. Physician's Approval Form
6. Agreement and Release of Liability Form
7. Informed Consent Agreement
8. Informed Consent for Participation in a Personal Fitness Training Program for Apparently Healthy Adults (Without Known or Suspected Heart Disease)
9. Informed Consent for Exercise Testing of Apparently Healthy Adults (Without Known or Suspected Heart Disease)
10. Informed Consent for Participation in an Exercise Program for Apparently Healthy Adults (Without Known or Suspected Heart Disease)
11. Express Assumption of Risk Form
12. Physician's Release for Activity Form
13. Guest Agreement and Waiver With Brief Medical History
14. Emergency Medical Authorization Form
15. Fitness Evaluation Form
16. Fitness Integration Tracking Form
17. Cardiovascular Assessment Data Sheet
18. Release of Information Form
19. Progress Notes
20. Incident Report Form
21. Theft Report Form
22. Special Event Sign-Up Sheet
23. Appointment Sheet
24. Sample Exercise Card
25. Physical Activity Readiness Medical Exam Form (PARmed-X)
26. Emergency Procedures Sheet
27. Health Questionnaire
28. Coronary Risk Factor Identification Form
29. Fitness Testing Form
30. Medical Clearance Form
31. Exercise Contract
32. Health, Fitness, and Racquet Sports Club Incident Report
33. Housekeeping Checklist—Fitness Equipment Room
34. Housekeeping Checklist—Locker Room

Physical Activity Readiness Questionnaire (PAR-Q)

Physical Activity Readiness
Questionnaire - PAR-Q
(revised 2002)

PAR-Q & YOU

(A Questionnaire for People Aged 15 to 69)

Regular physical activity is fun and healthy, and increasingly more people are starting to become more active every day. Being more active is very safe for most people. However, some people should check with their doctor before they start becoming much more physically active.

If you are planning to become much more physically active than you are now, start by answering the seven questions in the box below. If you are between the ages of 15 and 69, the PAR-Q will tell you if you should check with your doctor before you start. If you are over 69 years of age, and you are not used to being very active, check with your doctor.

Common sense is your best guide when you answer these questions. Please read the questions carefully and answer each one honestly: check YES or NO.

YES	NO		
☐	☐	1.	Has your doctor ever said that you have a heart condition <u>and</u> that you should only do physical activity recommended by a doctor?
☐	☐	2.	Do you feel pain in your chest when you do physical activity?
☐	☐	3.	In the past month, have you had chest pain when you were not doing physical activity?
☐	☐	4.	Do you lose your balance because of dizziness or do you ever lose consciousness?
☐	☐	5.	Do you have a bone or joint problem (for example, back, knee or hip) that could be made worse by a change in your physical activity?
☐	☐	6.	Is your doctor currently prescribing drugs (for example, water pills) for your blood pressure or heart condition?
☐	☐	7.	Do you know of <u>any other reason</u> why you should not do physical activity?

If you answered

YES to one or more questions

Talk with your doctor by phone or in person BEFORE you start becoming much more physically active or BEFORE you have a fitness appraisal. Tell your doctor about the PAR-Q and which questions you answered YES.

- You may be able to do any activity you want — as long as you start slowly and build up gradually. Or, you may need to restrict your activities to those which are safe for you. Talk with your doctor about the kinds of activities you wish to participate in and follow his/her advice.
- Find out which community programs are safe and helpful for you.

NO to all questions

If you answered NO honestly to <u>all</u> PAR-Q questions, you can be reasonably sure that you can:
- start becoming much more physically active – begin slowly and build up gradually. This is the safest and easiest way to go.
- take part in a fitness appraisal – this is an excellent way to determine your basic fitness so that you can plan the best way for you to live actively. It is also highly recommended that you have your blood pressure evaluated. If your reading is over 144/94, talk with your doctor before you start becoming much more physically active.

→

DELAY BECOMING MUCH MORE ACTIVE:
- if you are not feeling well because of a temporary illness such as a cold or a fever – wait until you feel better; or
- if you are or may be pregnant – talk to your doctor before you start becoming more active.

PLEASE NOTE: If your health changes so that you then answer YES to any of the above questions, tell your fitness or health professional. Ask whether you should change your physical activity plan.

<u>Informed Use of the PAR-Q:</u> The Canadian Society for Exercise Physiology, Health Canada, and their agents assume no liability for persons who undertake physical activity, and if in doubt after completing this questionnaire, consult your doctor prior to physical activity.

No changes permitted. You are encouraged to photocopy the PAR-Q but only if you use the entire form.

NOTE: If the PAR-Q is being given to a person before he or she participates in a physical activity program or a fitness appraisal, this section may be used for legal or administrative purposes.

"I have read, understood and completed this questionnaire. Any questions I had were answered to my full satisfaction."

NAME _____

SIGNATURE _____   DATE _____

SIGNATURE OF PARENT _____   WITNESS _____
or GUARDIAN (for participants under the age of majority)

Note: This physical activity clearance is valid for a maximum of 12 months from the date it is completed and becomes invalid if your condition changes so that you would answer YES to any of the seven questions.

CSEP
SCPE © Canadian Society for Exercise Physiology   Supported by: [🍁] Health Santé
                                                                              Canada Canada   continued on other side...

Form 2

Health History Questionnaire

Name _____   Company _____

Home address _____

Position _____

Telephone   home _____   work _____

Height _____   Weight _____

Gender _____   Birth date _____   Age _____

Regular physical activity is safe for most people. However, some individuals should check with their doctor before they start an exercise program. To help us determine if you should consult with your doctor before starting to exercise with (your organization), please read the following questions carefully and answer each one honestly. All information will be kept confidential. Please check YES or NO:

YES   NO

☐   ☐   1. Do you have a heart condition?

☐   ☐   2. Have you ever experienced a stroke?

☐   ☐   3. Do you have epilepsy?

☐   ☐   4. Are you pregnant?

☐   ☐   5. Do you have diabetes?

☐   ☐   6. Do you have emphysema?

☐   ☐   7. Do you feel pain in your chest when you engage in physical activity?

☐   ☐   8. Do you have chronic bronchitis?

☐   ☐   9. In the past month, have you had chest pain when you were not doing physical activity?

☐   ☐   10. Do you ever lose consciousness or do you ever lose control of your balance due to chronic dizziness?

☐   ☐   11. Are you currently being treated for a bone or joint problem that restricts you from engaging in physical activity?

☐   ☐   12. Has a physician ever told you or are you aware that you have high blood pressure?

☐   ☐   13. Has anyone in your immediate family (parents/brothers/sisters) had a heart attack, stroke, or cardiovascular disease before age 55?

☐   ☐   14. Has a physician ever told you or are you aware that you have a high cholesterol level?

☐   ☐   15. Do you currently smoke?

☐   ☐   16. Are you a male over 44 years of age?

☐   ☐   17. Are you a female over 54 years of age?

☐   ☐   18. Are you currently exercising *LESS* than 1 hour per week? If you answered no, please list your activities.

_____

☐   ☐   19. Are you currently taking any medication?

Please list the medication and its purpose _____

What are your specific fitness goals at (your organization)? (Indicate all that apply)

☐ Increase strength and endurance   ☐ Improve flexibility

☐ Improve cardiovascular fitness   ☐ Improve muscle tone

☐ Reduce body fat   ☐ Increase muscle mass

☐ Exercise regularly   ☐ Injury rehabilitation

☐ Sports conditioning   ☐ Other _____

What are your specific health goals at (your organization)? (Indicate all that apply)

☐ Reduce stress   ☐ Improve nutritional habits

☐ Control blood pressure   ☐ Control cholesterol

☐ Stop smoking   ☐ Achieve balance in life

☐ Improve productivity   ☐ Reduce back pain

☐ Feel better overall   ☐ Increase my health awareness

☐ Other (please be specific) _____

What motivated you to join (your organization)? (Indicate all that apply)

☐ Convenience/location

☐ Membership promotion

☐ Attended a (your organization) health promotion event at work

☐ Peer support

☐ Medical reasons

☐ Tried (your organization) as a guest

☐ Corporate membership

☐ Other _____

I have read, understood, and completed this questionnaire. Any questions that I had were answered to my full satisfaction.

Name _____ Date _____

Signature _____

STAFF USE ONLY

Cleared to exercise _____ Not cleared to exercise _____

Reason _____

Staff Signature _____ Date _____

Resting Heart Rate _____

Resting Blood Pressure _____

EP _____

Reprinted, by permission, from Fitcorp, 1990, *Fitcorp program manual* (Boston, MA: Fitcorp).

Form 3
Guest Health History Questionnaire

Name _____ Date _____

Date of birth _____

Employer _____

Title _____

Home address _____ City _____ Zip _____

Phone (home) _____ (work) _____

Gender   (Please circle)   M   F

Guest of _____

Health insurance provider _____

In case of emergency contact _____

Regular physical activity is safe for most people. However, some individuals should check with their doctor before they start an exercise program. To help us determine if you should consult with your doctor before starting to exercise with (your organization), please read the following questions carefully and answer each one honestly. All information will be kept confidential. Please check YES or NO:

YES NO

☐ ☐ 1. Do you have a heart condition?

☐ ☐ 2. Have you ever experienced a stroke?

☐ ☐ 3. Do you have epilepsy?

☐ ☐ 4. Are you pregnant?

☐ ☐ 5. Do you have diabetes?

☐ ☐ 6. Do you have emphysema?

☐ ☐ 7. Do you feel pain in your chest when you engage in physical activity?

☐ ☐ 8. Do you have chronic bronchitis?

☐ ☐ 9. In the past month, have you had chest pain when you were not doing physical activity?

☐ ☐ 10. Do you ever lose consciousness or do you ever lose control of your balance due to chronic dizziness?

☐ ☐ 11. Are you currently being treated for a bone or joint problem that restricts you from engaging in physical activity?

☐ ☐ 12. Has a physician ever told you or are you aware that you have high blood pressure?

☐ ☐ 13. Has anyone in your immediate family (parents/brothers/sisters) had a heart attack, stroke, or cardiovascular disease before age 55?

☐ ☐ 14. Has a physician ever told you or are you aware that you have a high cholesterol level?

☐ ☐ 15. Do you currently smoke?

YES NO

☐ ☐   16. Are you a male over 44 years of age?

☐ ☐   17. Are you a female over 54 years of age?

☐ ☐   18. Are you currently exercising *LESS* than 1 hour per week? If you answered no, please list your activities.

_____

☐ ☐   19. Are you currently taking any medication? Please list the medication and its purpose.

_____

How did you hear about (your organization)?

_____ Employer   _____ Yellow Pages   _____ Friend

_____ Television   _____ Newspaper   _____ Radio

_____ Co-worker   _____ Health ins. plan   _____ Worksite event

Are you interested in joining (your organization)?   Y or N

Are you interested in learning how (your organization) can develop a corporate fitness and wellness benefit for your organization?   Y or N

I understand that any exercise program I undertake may create physical stress and subsequent harmful effects. I agree that it is solely my responsibility and not the responsibility of (your organization) to require me to consult with a physician prior to commencing any exercise program, to remain under medical supervision if that is indicated, and to seek medical assistance in the event of an injury. I recognize that the use of the equipment entails some risk of accidental injury to myself and to others and I agree that I will use such equipment and facilities with due care.

Signature _____   Date _____

STAFF USE ONLY

☐ **Cleared to exercise**   ☐ **Not cleared to exercise**   ☐ **Guest #** _____

Reason _____

Staff Signature _____   **Date** _____

Visit Date/Time _____   **Visit Date/Time** _____

Visit Date/Time _____   **Visit Date/Time** _____

Visit Date/Time _____   **Visit Date/Time** _____

Reprinted, by permission, from Fitcorp, 1990, *Fitcorp program manual* (Boston, MA: Fitcorp).

Form 4
Physician's Statement and Clearance Form

At (your organization), your safety is our primary concern. For that reason, we comply with the health and fitness standards of the American College of Sports Medicine and the International Health, Racquet and Sportsclub Association.

On the Health History Questionnaire you just completed, you identified that you have one or more coronary and/or other medical risk factors that may impair your ability to exercise safely. For this reason, you need to have a physician complete and return this medical clearance form before you can begin exercising at (your organization).

We recognize that you are eager to start your fitness program, and we sincerely regret any inconvenience that this may cause you. However, please keep in mind that we want your exercise experience at (your organization) to be as safe as possible.

In order to expedite this process, we will gladly fax this form directly to the physician of your choice. If the doctor is aware of your medical history, he/she may be able to complete this form and fax it right back to us. In many cases the delay is only one day.

I hereby give my physician permission to release any pertinent medical information from any medical records to the staff at (your organization). All information will be kept confidential.

Patient's signature _____ Date _____

Information requested for _____

Reason for medical clearance _____

Physician's name _____

Phone _____ Fax _____

Address _____

For Physician Use Only

Please check one of the following statements:

_____ I concur with my patient's participation with no restrictions.

_____ I concur with my patient's participation in an exercise program if he/she restricts activities to:

_____

_____ I do not concur with my patient's participation in an exercise program (if checked, the individual will not be allowed to join [your organization]).

Reason
_____

Physician's name (type or print) _____

Physician's signature _____ Date _____

Please return fax to: General Manager _____

Phone _____ **Fax** _____

Reprinted, by permission, from Fitcorp 1990, *Fitcorp program manual* (Boston, MA: Fitcorp).

Form 5

Physician's Approval Form

_____ has medical approval to participate in fitness

programs and in the use of exercise equipment at various sites, including home or office, that may be pro-

vided by and/or recommended by_____ .

The following restrictions apply (if none, so state): _____

_____

_____

_____

_____

_____

Physician's signature

_____

Physician's name

_____

Street address

_____ _____ _____

City   State   Zip

_____

Phone

_____

Date

*** Please attach a copy of the results of the latest physical examination.

Note. The law varies from state to state. No form should be adopted or used by any program without individualized legal advice.

Reprinted, by permission from B.E. Koeberle, 1990, *Legal aspects of personal fitness training* (Canton, OH: Professional Reports Corporation), 145.

Form 6

Agreement and Release of Liability Form

1. In consideration of gaining membership or being allowed to participate in the activities and programs of _____ and to use its facilities, equipment, and machinery in addition to the payment of any fee or charge, I do hereby waive, release and forever discharge _____ and its officers, agents, employees, representatives, executors, and all others from any and all responsibilities or liability for injuries or damages resulting from my participation in any activities or my use of equipment or machinery in the above-mentioned facilities or arising out of my participation in any activities at said facility. I do also hereby release all of those mentioned and any others acting upon their behalf from any responsibility or liability for any injury or damage to myself, including those caused by the negligent act or omission of any of those mentioned or others acting on their behalf or in any way arising out of or connected with my participation in any activities of _____ or the use of any equipment at _____ . (**Please initial** _____)

2. I understand and am aware that strength, feasibility, and aerobic exercise, including the use of equipment, is a potentially hazardous activity. I also understand that fitness activities involve a risk of injury and even death and that I am voluntarily participating in these activities and using equipment and machinery with knowledge of the dangers involved. I hereby agree to expressly assume and accept any and all risks of injury or death. (**Please initial** _____)

3. I do hereby further declare myself to be physically sound and suffering from no condition, impairment, disease, infirmity, or other illness that would prevent my participation in any of the activities and programs of _____ or use of equipment or machinery except as hereinafter stated. I do hereby acknowledge that I have been informed of the need for a physician's approval for my participation in an exercise/fitness activity or in the use of exercise equipment and machinery. I also acknowledge that it has been recommended that I have a yearly or more frequent physical examination and consultation with my physician as to physical activity, exercise, and use of exercise and training equipment so that I might have recommendations concerning these fitness activities and equipment use. I acknowledge that I have either had a physical examination and have been given a physician's permission to participate, or that I have decided to participate in activity and/or use of equipment and machinery without the approval of my physician and do hereby assume all responsibility for my participation and activities, and utilization of equipment and machinery in my activities. (**Please initial** _____)

Date _____ Signature _____

Note. The law varies from state to state. No form should be adopted or used by any program without individualized legal advice.

Reprinted, by permission from D Herbert, 1989, "Avoiding allegations of misrepresentation/fraud in program documents," *The Exercise Standards and Malpractice Reporter* 3(2):30-31.

Form 7

Informed Consent Agreement

Thank you for choosing to use the facilities, services, or programs of _____. We request your understanding and cooperation in maintaining both your and our safety and health by reading and signing the following informed consent agreement.

I, _____, declare that I intend to use some or all of the activities, facilities, programs, and services offered by _____ and I understand that each person, myself included, has a different capacity for participating in such activities, facilities, programs, and services. I am aware that all activities, services, and programs offered are either educational, recreational, or self-directed in nature. I assume full responsibility, during and after my participation, for my choices to use or apply, at my own risk, any portion of the information or instruction I receive.

I understand that part of the risk involved in undertaking any activity or program is relative to my own state of fitness or health (physical, mental, or emotional) and to the awareness, care, and skill with which I conduct myself in that activity or program. I acknowledge that my choice to participate in any activity, service, and program of _____ brings with it my assumption of those risks or results stemming from this choice and the fitness, health, awareness, care, and skill that I possess and use.

I further understand that the activities, programs, and services offered by _____ are sometimes conducted by personnel who may not be licensed, certified, or registered instructors or professionals. I accept the fact that the skills and competencies of some employees and/or volunteers will vary according to their training and experience and that no claim is made to offer assessment or treatment of any mental or physical disease or condition by those who are not duly licensed, certified, or registered and herein employed to provide such professional services.

I recognize that by participating in the activities, facilities, programs, and services offered by _____, I may experience potential health risks such as transient light-headedness, fainting, abnormal blood pressure, chest discomfort, leg cramps, and nausea and that I assume willfully those risks. I acknowledge my obligation to immediately inform the nearest supervising employee of any pain, discomfort, fatigue, or any other symptoms that I may suffer during and immediately after my participation. I understand that I may stop or delay my participation in any activity or procedure if I so desire and that I may also be requested to stop and rest by a supervising employee who observes any symptoms of distress or abnormal response.

I understand that I may ask any questions or request further explanation or information about the activities, facilities, programs, and services offered by _____ at any time before, during, or after my participation.

I declare that I have read, understood, and agree to the contents of this informed consent agreement in its entirety.

Signature _____

Date of signing _____

Witness _____

Note. The law varies from state to state. No form should be adopted or used by any program without individualized legal advice.

> ## *Form 8*
>
> # Informed Consent for Participation in a Personal Fitness Training Program for Apparently Healthy Adults
>
> (Without Known or Suspected Heart Disease)

Name _____

1. PURPOSE AND EXPLANATION OF PROCEDURE

I hereby consent to voluntarily engage in an acceptable plan of personal fitness training. I also give consent to be placed in personal fitness training program activities that are recommended to me for improvement of my general health and well-being. These may include dietary counseling, stress management, and health/fitness education activities. The levels of exercise I perform will be based on my cardiorespiratory (heart and lungs) and muscular fitness. I understand that I may be required to undergo a graded exercise test as well as other fitness tests prior to the start of my personal fitness training program in order to evaluate and assess my present level of fitness. I will be given exact personal instructions regarding the amount and kind of exercise I should do. I agree to participate 3 times per week in the formal program sessions. Professionally trained personal fitness trainers will provide leadership to direct my activities, monitor my performance, and otherwise evaluate my effort. Depending on my health status, I may or may not be required to have my blood pressure and heart rate evaluated during these sessions to regulate my exercise within desired limits. I understand that I am expected to attend every session and to follow staff instructions with regard to exercise, diet, stress management, and other health/fitness-related programs. If I am taking prescribed medications, I have already so informed the program staff and further agree to so inform them promptly of any changes my doctor or I make with regard to use of these. I will be given the opportunity for periodic assessment and evaluation at regular intervals after the start of my program.

I have been informed that during my participation in this personal fitness training program, I will be asked to complete the physical activities unless symptoms such as fatigue, shortness of breath, chest discomfort, or similar occurrences appear. At that point, I have been advised that it is my complete right to decrease or stop exercise and that it is my obligation to inform the personal fitness training program personnel of my symptoms. I hereby state that I have been so advised and agree to inform the personal fitness training program personnel of my symptoms, should any develop.

I understand that while I exercise, a personal fitness trainer will periodically monitor my performance and perhaps measure my pulse and blood pressure or assess my feelings of effort for the purposes of monitoring my progress. I also understand that the personal fitness trainer may reduce or stop my exercise program when any of these findings so indicate that this should be done for my safety and benefit.

I also understand that during the performance of my personal fitness training program, physical touching and positioning of my body may be necessary to assess my muscular and bodily reactions to specific exercises, as well as ensure that I am using proper technique and body alignment. I expressly consent to the physical contact for these reasons.

2. RISKS

I understand and have been informed that there exists the remote possibility of adverse changes occurring during exercise including, but not limited to, abnormal blood pressure, fainting, dizziness, disorders of heart rhythm, and very rare instances of heart attack, stroke, or even death. I further understand and I have been informed that there exists the risk of bodily injury including, but not limited to, injuries to the muscles, ligaments, tendons, and joints of the body. I have been told that every effort will be made to minimize these occurrences by proper staff assessments of my condition before each exercise session, by staff supervision during exercise, and by my own careful control of exercise efforts. I fully understand the risks associated with exercise, including the risk of bodily injury, heart attack, stroke, or even death, but knowing these risks, it is my desire to participate as herein indicated.

3. BENEFITS TO BE EXPECTED AND AVAILABLE ALTERNATIVES TO EXERCISE

I understand that this program may or may not benefit my physical fitness or general health. I recognize that involvement in the exercise sessions and personal fitness training sessions will allow me to learn proper ways to perform conditioning exercises, use fitness equipment, and regulate physical effort. These experiences should benefit me by indicating how my physical limitations may affect my ability to perform various physical activities. I further understand that if I closely follow the program's instructions, I will likely improve my exercise capacity and fitness level after a period of 3 to 6 months.

4. CONFIDENTIALITY AND USE OF INFORMATION

I have been informed that the information obtained in this personal fitness training program will be treated as privileged and confidential and will consequently not be released or revealed to any person without my express written consent. I do, however, agree to the use of any information that is not personally identifiable with me for research and statistical purposes so long as same does not identify me or provide facts that could lead to my identification. I also agree to the use of any information for the purpose of consultation with other health/fitness professionals, including my doctor. Any other information obtained, however, will be used by the program staff in the course of prescribing exercise for me and evaluating my progress in the program.

5. INQUIRIES AND FREEDOM OF CONSENT

I have been given an opportunity to ask certain questions as to the procedures of this program. Generally, these requests have been noted by the interviewing staff with his/her responses as follows:

_____

_____

_____

I further understand that there are also other remote risks that may be associated with this personal fitness training program. Despite the fact that a complete accounting of all these remote risks has not been provided to me, it is still my desire to participate.

I acknowledge that I have read this document in its entirety or that it has been read to me if I have been unable to read same.

I expressly consent to the rendition of all services and procedures as explained herein by all program personnel.

Date _____

_____

Client's signature

By _____
Authorized representative

Note. The law varies from state to state. No form should be adopted or used by any program without individualized legal advice.

Reprinted, by permission from B.E. Koeberle, 1990, *Legal aspects of personal fitness training* (Canton, OH: Professional Reports Corporation), 149-151.

> ## *Form 9*
> # Informed Consent for Exercise Testing of Apparently Healthy Adults
> ### (Without Known or Suspected Heart Disease)

Name _____

1. PURPOSE AND EXPLANATION OF TEST

I hereby consent to voluntarily engage in an exercise test to determine my circulatory and respiratory fitness. I also consent to the taking of samples of my exhaled air during exercise to properly measure my oxygen consumption. I also consent, if necessary, to have a small blood sample drawn by needle from my arm for blood chemistry analysis and to the performance of lung function and body fat (skinfold pinch) tests. It is my understanding that the information obtained will help me evaluate future physical activities and sports activities in which I may engage.

Before I undergo the test, I certify to the program that I am in good health and have had a physical examination conducted by a licensed medical physician within the last _____ months. Further, I hereby represent and inform the program that I have completed the pretest history interview presented to me by the program staff and have provided correct responses to the questions as indicated on the history form or as supplied to the interviewer. It is my understanding that I will be interviewed by a physician or other person prior to my undergoing the test who will in the course of interviewing me determine if there are any reasons which would make it undesirable or unsafe for me to take the test. Consequently, I understand that it is important that I provide complete and accurate responses to the interviewer and recognize that my failure to do so could lead to possible unnecessary injury to myself during the test.

The test I will undergo will be performed on a motor-driven treadmill or bicycle ergometer with the amount of effort gradually increasing. As I understand it, this increase in effort will continue until I feel and verbally report to the operator any symptoms such as fatigue, shortness of breath, or chest discomfort which may appear. It is my understanding and I have been clearly advised that it is my right to request that a test be stopped at any point if I feel unusual discomfort or fatigue. I have been advised that I should immediately upon experiencing any such symptoms, or if I so choose, inform the operator that I wish to stop the test at that or any other point. My wishes in this regard shall be absolutely carried out.

It is further my understanding that prior to beginning the test, I will be connected by electrodes and cables to an electrocardiographic recorder, which will enable the program personnel to monitor my cardiac (heart) activity. It is my understanding that during the test itself, a trained observer will monitor my responses continuously and take frequent readings of blood pressure, the electrocardiogram, and my expressed feelings of effort. I realize that a true determination of my exercise capacity depends on progressing the test to the point of my fatigue.

Once the test has been completed, but before I am released from the test area, I will be given special instructions about showering and recognition of certain symptoms that may appear within the first 24 hours after the test. I agree to follow these instructions and promptly contact the program personnel or medical providers if such symptoms develop.

2. RISKS

I understand and have been informed that there exists the possibility of adverse changes during the actual test. I have been informed that these changes could include abnormal blood pressure, fainting, disorders of heart rhythm, stroke, and very rare instances of heart attack or even death. I have been told that every effort will be made to minimize these occurrences by preliminary examination and by precautions and observations taken during the test. I have also been informed that emergency equipment and personnel are readily available to deal with these unusual situations should they occur. I understand that there is a risk of injury, heart attack, or even death as a result of my performance of this test, but knowing those risks, it is my desire to proceed to take the test as herein indicated.

3. BENEFITS TO BE EXPECTED AND AVAILABLE ALTERNATIVES TO THE EXERCISE TESTING PROCEDURE

The results of this test may or may not benefit me. Potential benefits relate mainly to my personal motives for taking the test, that is, knowing my exercise capacity in relation to the general population, understanding my fitness for certain sports and recreational activities, planning my physical conditioning program, or evaluating the effects of my recent physical activity habits. Although my fitness might also be evaluated by alternative means, for example, a bench step test or an outdoor running test, such tests do not provide as accurate a fitness assessment as the treadmill or bike test nor do those options allow equally effective monitoring of my responses.

4. CONFIDENTIALITY AND USE OF INFORMATION

I have been informed that the information obtained in this exercise test will be treated as privileged and confidential and will consequently not be released or revealed to any person without my express written consent. I do, however, agree to the use of any information for research or statistical purposes so long as same does not provide facts that could lead to my identification. Any other information obtained, however, will be used only by the program staff to evaluate my exercise status or needs.

5. INQUIRIES AND FREEDOM OF CONSENT

I have been given an opportunity to ask certain questions as to the procedures. Generally these requests, which have been noted by the testing staff, and their responses are as follows:

_____

_____

_____

I further understand that there are also other remote risks that may be associated with this procedure. Despite the fact that a complete accounting of all these remote risks has not been provided to me, I still desire to proceed with the test.

I acknowledge that I have read this document in its entirety or that it has been read to me if I have been unable to read same.

I consent to the rendition of all services and procedures as explained herein by all program personnel.

Date _____

_____

Participant's signature

_____

Witness' signature

_____

Test supervisor's signature

Note. The law varies from state to state. No form should be adopted or used by any program without individualized legal advice.

Reprinted, by permission, from D. Herbert, 1994, _Legal aspects of sports medicine_, 2nd ed. (Canton, OH: Professional Reports Corporation).

> ## Form 10
>
> # Informed Consent for Participation in an Exercise Program for Apparently Healthy Adults
>
> ## (Without Known or Suspected Heart Disease)

Name _____

1. PURPOSE AND EXPLANATION OF PROCEDURE

I hereby consent to voluntarily engage in an acceptable plan of exercise conditioning. I also give consent to be placed in program activities that are recommended to me for improvement of my general health and well-being. These may include dietary counseling, stress reduction, and health education activities. The levels of exercise I will perform will be based upon my cardiorespiratory (heart and lungs) fitness as determined through my recent laboratory graded exercise evaluation. I will be given exact instructions regarding the amount and kind of exercise I should do. I agree to participate 3 times per week in the formal program sessions. Professionally trained personnel will provide leadership to direct my activities, monitor my performance, and otherwise evaluate my effort. Depending upon my health status, I may or may not be required to have my blood pressure and heart rate evaluated during these sessions to regulate my exercise within desired limits. I understand that I am expected to attend every session and to follow staff instructions with regard to exercise, diet, stress management, and smoking cessation. If I am taking prescribed medications, I have already so informed the program staff and further agree to so inform them promptly of any changes my doctor or I make with regard to use of these. I will be given the opportunity for periodic assessment with laboratory evaluations at 6 months after the start of my program. Should I remain in the program thereafter, additional evaluations will generally be given at 12 month intervals. The program may change the foregoing schedule of evaluations, if this is considered desirable for health reasons.

I have been informed that during my participation in exercise, I will be asked to complete the physical activities unless symptoms such as fatigue, shortness of breath, chest discomfort, or similar occurrences appear. At that point, I have been advised it is my complete right to decrease or stop exercise and that it is my obligation to inform the program personnel of my symptoms. I hereby state that I have been so advised and agree to inform the program personnel of my symptoms, should any develop.

I understand that, while I exercise, a trained observer will periodically monitor my performance and perhaps measure my pulse and blood pressure or assess my feelings of effort for the purposes of monitoring my progress. I also understand that the observer may reduce or stop my exercise program when any of these findings so indicate that this should be done for my safety and benefit.

2. RISKS

I understand and have been informed that there exists the remote possibility during exercise of adverse changes including abnormal blood pressure, fainting, disorders of heart rhythm, and very rare instances of heart attack or even death. I have been told that every effort will be made to minimize these occurrences by proper staff assessment of my condition before each exercise session, by staff supervision during exercise, and by my own careful control of exercise efforts. I have also been informed that emergency equipment and personnel are readily available to deal with unusual situations should these occur. I understand that there is a risk of injury, heart attack, or even death as a result of my exercise, but knowing those risks, I desire to participate as herein indicated.

3. BENEFITS TO BE EXPECTED AND ALTERNATIVES AVAILABLE TO EXERCISE

I understand that this program may or may not benefit my physical fitness or general health. I recognize that involvement in the exercise sessions will allow me to learn proper ways to perform conditioning exercises, use fitness equipment, and regulate physical effort. These experiences should benefit me by indicating how my physical limitations may affect my ability to perform various physical activities. I further understand that if I closely follow the program instructions, I will likely improve my exercise capacity after a period of 3 to 6 months.

4. CONFIDENTIALITY AND USE OF INFORMATION

I have been informed that the information obtained in this exercise program will be treated as privileged and confidential and will consequently not be released or revealed to any person without my express written consent. I do, however, agree to the use of any information that is not personally identifiable with me for research and statistical purposes so long as same does not identify me or provide facts that could lead to my identification. Any other information obtained, however, will be used only by the program staff in the course of prescribing exercise for me and evaluating my progress in the program.

5. INQUIRIES AND FREEDOM OF CONSENT

I have been given an opportunity to ask certain questions as to the procedures of this program. Generally these requests have been noted by the interviewing staff member, and his/her responses are as follows.

_____

_____

_____

I further understand that there are also other remote risks that may be associated with this program. Despite the fact that a complete accounting of all these remote risks has not been provided to me, I still desire to participate.

I acknowledge that I have read this document in its entirety or that it has been read to me if I have been unable to read same.

I consent to the rendition of all services and procedures as explained herein by all program personnel.

Date _____

_____
Participant's signature

_____
Witness' signature

_____
Test supervisor's signature

Note. The law varies from state to state. No form should be adopted or used by any program without individualized legal advice.

Reprinted, by permission, from D. Herbert, 1994, _Legal aspects of sports medicine_, 2nd ed. (Canton, OH: Professional Reports Corporation).

Form 11

Express Assumption of Risk Form

I, the undersigned, hereby expressly and affirmatively state that I wish to participate in _____. I realize that my participation in this activity involves risks of injury, including but not limited to _____ (list) _____ and even the possibility of death. I also recognize that there are many other risks of injury, including serious disabling injuries, that may arise due to my participation in this activity and that it is not possible to specifically list each and every individual injury risk. However, knowing the material risks and appreciating, knowing, and reasonably anticipating that other injuries and even death are a possibility, I hereby expressly assume all of the delineated risks of injury, all other possible risk of injury, and even risk of death, which could occur by reason of my participation.

I have had an opportunity to ask questions. Any questions I have asked have been answered to my complete satisfaction. I subjectively understand the risks of my participation in this activity, and knowing and appreciating these risks, I voluntarily choose to participate, assuming all risks of injury or even death due to my participation.

_____   _____
Witness   Participant

_____
Dated

Notes of questions and answers

_____
_____
_____

This is, as stated, a true and accurate record of what was asked and answered.

_____
Participant

To be checked by program staff	*Checked*	*Initials*
I. Risks were orally discussed.	_____	_____
II. Questions were asked, and the participant indicated complete understanding of the risks.	_____	_____
III. Questions were not asked, but an opportunity to ask questions was provided and the participant indicated complete understanding of the risks.	_____	_____

_____   _____
Staff member   Dated

Note. The law varies from state to state. No form should be adopted or used by any program without individualized legal advice.

Reprinted, by permission, from D. Herbert, 1994, "Avoiding allegations of misrepresentation/fraud in program documents," *The Exercise Standards and Malpractice Reporter* 3(2): 30-31.

Form 12

Physician's Release for Activity Form

_____ has recently enrolled for membership at East Side/West Side Athletic Clubs. The club membership includes two complimentary orientation sessions with our qualified fitness professionals (degreed and/or certified in the field), as well as the opportunity to participate in numerous group fitness classes and individual programs.

On completion of the PAR-Q (Physical Activity Readiness Questionnaire), it has been determined that this new member is best served by additional or supplemental recommendations by his/her Care Provider.

Please take the time to review your client's medical history and the PAR-Q accompanied with this request. If he/she can be released for physical activity, please complete the information below and let us know if there are any modifications or special needs.

Member's signature for release of information _____

Date _____

Club staff faxing this information (print name) _____

As a physician, it is my understanding that the person listed above wishes to participate in physical activity at the Club and has been referred to myself (his/her physician) before beginning a regular program. **Here are my specific recommendations and/or comments regarding this new member and his/her involvement in an exercise program:**

Physician's printed name _____

Date _____

Physician's signature _____

Form 13

Guest Agreement and Waiver With Brief Medical History

Date _____

Name _____

Company name _____

Mailing address _____

City _____ State _____ Zip _____

Phone: (W) _____ (H) _____

Guest of: _____

Please answer the following seven questions

YES NO

☐ ☐ 1. Has your doctor ever said you have heart trouble?

☐ ☐ 2. Do you frequently have pains in your heart and chest?

☐ ☐ 3. Do you often feel faint or have spells of severe dizziness?

☐ ☐ 4. Has a doctor ever said your blood pressure was too high?

☐ ☐ 5. Has you doctor ever told you that you have a bone or joint problem such as arthritis that has been aggravated by exercise or might be made worse by exercise?

☐ ☐ 6. Is there any good physical reason not mentioned here why you should not follow an activity program even if you wanted to?

☐ ☐ 7. Are you over age 65 and not accustomed to vigorous exercise?

Guest Agreement/Waiver

The undersigned guest agrees to abide by the rules of the Club, including the completion of the above medical questionnaire.

The undersigned guest agrees that all use of the Club's facilities, services and programs shall be undertaken at his/her sole risk and the Club shall not be liable for any injuries, accidents or deaths occurring to guest, arising either directly or indirectly out of utilizing the Club's facilities, services and programs. The guest, for him/herself and on behalf of his/her executors, administrators, heirs and assigns, does hereby expressly release, discharge, waive, relinquish, and covenants not to sue Club, it officers and agents for all such claims, demands, injuries, damages or cause of action, with respect to use of the Club's facilities, programs and services.

The undersigned guest declares that he/she has completed the enclosed medical questionnaire as required by the Club and that he/she declares he/she is physically able to participate in physical activity. Furthermore, guest declares that the Club has advised guest to obtain a medical clearance in the event he/she answer yes to any of the medical history questions, or if he/she is unsure of his/her physical health and that guest maintains that he/she is physically capable of pursuing physical activity in the Club without such steps being taken or has done so.

Guest signature _____

Date _____

Form 14

Emergency Medical Authorization Form

I/we, the undersigned, am/are the father and mother of _____ minor(s).

CONSENT

I/we hereby give consent, in the event I/we cannot be contacted within a reasonable time, for (1) the administration of any treatment deemed necessary for my/our children by Dr. _____, or any of his/her associates, the preferred physician, or Dr. _____, or any of his/her associates, the preferred dentist, or in the event the appropriate preferred practitioner is not available, by another licensed, qualified physician or dentist; and (2) the transfer of any of my/our children to _____ Hospital, the preferred hospital, or any hospital reasonably accessible.

MAJOR SURGERY

This authorization does not cover nonemergency major surgery unless the medical opinions of two other licensed physicians or dentists concurring in the necessity for such surgery are obtained prior to the performance of such surgery and unless all reasonable attempts to contact me/us have been unsuccessful, defining such period for nonemergency surgery as 24 hours.

MEDICAL DATA

The following is needed by any hospital or practitioner not having access to my/our children's medical history:

Allergies: _____

Medication being taken: _____

Physical impairments: _____

Other pertinent facts to which physician should be alerted: _____

Medical insurance coverage: _____

I/we, the undersigned parent(s), also do by these premises appoint and constitute _____ and _____ and/or _____ as temporary custodians of my/our children above mentioned, for the period of _____, 20 ____, through and including _____, 20 ____, and do hereby authorize them to obtain any X-ray examination, anesthesia, medical or surgical diagnosis or treatment, and hospital care to be rendered to my/our children in our absence, under the general or special supervision, and on the advice of, a licensed physician, surgeon, anesthesiologist, dentist, or other qualified personnel acting under their supervision.

Witnesses _____

_____

State of _____

SS: _____

_____ County

Note. The law varies from state to state. No form should be adopted or used by any program without individualized legal advice.

Form 15

Fitness Evaluation Form

Date _____ / _____ / _____

Member name _____ Membership number _____

Member address _____ City _____ State _____ (Zip) _____ Member phone number _____

Physician's name _____

Physician's address _____ City _____ State _____ (Zip) _____ Physician's phone number _____

I.   General physiological information   Birthdate _____ / _____ / _____
    1. Age _____ 2. Sex M ☐ F ☐ 3. Risk category _____ 4. Height _____ ft _____ in.
    5. Weight _____ 6. RHR _____ 7. RBP _____ 8. Predicted Max HR _____
    Medications_____ _____
    Exercise history _____

II. Cardiovascular assessment
    1. RHR supine_____
    2. RBP supine _____
    3. RBP standing _____
    4. Predicted heart rate

                Max _____
                90% _____
                80% _____
                70% _____

    5. HVHR _____
    Protocol _____
    Equipment _____
    Max HR _____ Max BP _____/_____
    Max met _____

Stage	Time	Speed KPM	Grade	HR	BP	DP	ST	Comments
1	1							
	2							
	3							
2	1							
	2							
	3							
3	1							
	2							
	3							
4	1							
	2							
	3							
5	1							
	2							
	3							
Rest	1							
	3							
	6							
	9							

III. Lung capacity
    1. Vital capacity ___/___% Pred.
    2. FEV   ___/___% Pred.

IV. Flexibility
    1. Sit'n'reach ___ ___ ___ in.

V.   Muscular strength and endurance
    1. Grip ____/____/____ KgR ____/____/____ KgL
    2. Trunk curl/sit-up _____ # _____ Time
    3. _____ _____

VI. Body composition
    A. Skin folds   1   2   Avg.
        1. Chest   _____ _____ _____
        2. Subscapula   _____ _____ _____
        3. Suprailliac _____ _____ _____
        4. Umbilical   _____ _____ _____
        5. Tricep   _____ _____ _____
        6. Ant. thigh   _____ _____ _____
                Total skin folds   _____

    B. Body fat
        1. Percent fat _____ %
        2. Fat wt. _____ lb
        3. Lean wt. _____ lb
        4. Ideal percent fat _____ %
        5. Ideal wt. _____ lb

    C. Girths
        1. Neck   _____
        2. Shoulder _____
        3. Chest   _____
        4. Waist   _____
        5. Hips   _____
        6. Thigh ___ R ___ L
        7. Calf   ___ R ___ L
        8. Bicep ___ R ___ L
        9. Forearm ___ R ___ L

VII. Blood chemistry
    1. Cholesterol _____
    2. Chol./HDL _____
    3. LDL/HDL _____
    4. Triglycerides _____
    5. Glucose _____
    6. Hematocrit _____

Note: RHR = resting heart rate; RBP = resting blood pressure; MET = unit of metabolic measurement; HVHR = hyperventilating heart rate; FEV = forced expiratory volume; HR = heart rate; BP = blood pressure; DP = double product; ST = S-T segment; KgR = kilogram right hand; KgL = kilogram left hand. The law varies from state to state. No form should be adopted or used by any program without individualized legal advice.

Form 16

Fitness Integration Tracking Form

Member's name _____ Age _____ Acct.# _____ Acct. type _____

Consultation appt. Date/time _____ Fit specialist _____ Coach _____

REASONS

(check)   (rank)

☐ Lose body fat   _____
☐ Stress release   _____
☐ Meet similar folk   _____
☐ Family recreation   _____
☐ Strengthen/Tone   _____
☐ Self-esteem increase   _____
☐ Energy level increase _____
☐ _____   _____

INTERESTS

☐ Lose body fat   ☐ Karate   ☐ Personal training
☐ Weight training   ☐ Massage   ☐ Child care
☐ Swimming   ☐ Water exercise classes ☐ Physical therapy
☐ Exercise group classes ☐ Fitness evaluation   ☐ Nutrition
☐ Youth activities   ☐ Swim lessons   ☐ Social events
☐ Racquetball   ☐ Sports leagues   ☐ Volleyball
☐ Basketball   ☐ Fitness leagues   ☐ _____
☐ Sauna/steam   ☐ Jacuzzi   ☐ _____

SUCCESS PLAN

1. My MAIN objective is: _____

2. Why? _____

3. How will this accomplishment make you feel? _____

4. When would you like to accomplish this? _____

5. Why by then? _____

6. Baby Steps: _____

7. Will you need support in accomplishing these steps or changes? yes/no

   From whom? (family, training coach, social group, work peers, etc.) _____

8. What days of the week do you see yourself using the Club (circle) S   M   T   W   Th   F   S

9. Time of day? _____ # of Club visits per week?_____

10. Are #8 and #9 above realistic for you?   yes/no _____

11. If you consistently follow through on Baby Steps, how will you feel? _____

12. Do you foresee any potential obstacle or distractions? _____

13. How can I assist you in accomplishing your goals?_____

14. What type of coaching/support would benefit you most?

    _____

15. Notes: _____

    _____

Form 17

Cardiovascular Assessment Data Sheet

Name _____ Date _____ Age _____

Weight (kg) _____ Resting heart rate _____

Age-predicted max heart rate

60% _____ 65% _____ 70% _____ 90% _____

Mode of cardiovascular evaluation: bike RPMs _____, treadmill (please circle one)

   I. Warm-up workload: _____

       1 min _____   RPE _____

       2 min _____   BP _____

       3 min _____

       4 min _____

  II. Target workload #1: _____

       1 min _____   RPE _____

       2 min _____   BP _____

       3 min _____

       4 min _____

 III. Target workload #2 (if indicated): _____

       1 min _____   RPE _____

       2 min _____   BP _____

       3 min _____

       4 min _____

 IV. Cool-down workload: _____

       1 min _____   RPE _____

       2 min _____   BP _____

  V. $\dot{V}O_2$ max calculation conversion to METs:

      Predicted $\dot{V}O_2$ max (L/min) _____ × age factor _____ = maximum $\dot{V}O_2$ (L/min) _____

      $\dot{V}O_2$ max (ml/min) _____ – wt (kg) _____ = $\dot{V}O_2$max (ml/kg/min) _____

      $\dot{V}O_2$ max (ml/kg/min) _____ – 3.5 = predicted maximal capacity in METs

 VI. Summary

     • Predicted maximal capacity (METs) _____

     • Recommended training range (METs) _____

     • Recommended training range (heart rate) _____

Note. BP = blood pressure; MET = unit of metabolic measurement; RPM = rotations per minute; RPE = rate of perceived exertion.

Form 18

Release of Information Form

To whom it may concern:

Please be advised that (_____) and any member, associate, or designee of that firm is hereby authorized to inspect and copy or be furnished copies of any and all hospital, dental, or medical records of any sort as well as charts, notes, medical bills, dental bills, X-rays, lab reports, and prescriptions and is to be furnished any and all other information without limitations pertaining to any confinement, examination, treatment, or condition of myself, including medical, dental, psychological, or other treatment; examinations; or counseling for any medical, dental, or psychological condition.

This authorization shall be considered as continuing and you may rely on it in all respects unless you have previously been advised by me in writing to the contrary. It is expressly understood by the undersigned and you are hereby authorized to accept a copy or photocopy of this medical authorization with the same validity as though an original had been presented to you.

Dated this _____ day of _____, 20 _____.

X _____

Note. The law varies from state to state. No form should be adopted or used by any program without individualized legal advice.

Reprinted, by permission from B.E. Koeberle, 1990, *Legal aspects of personal fitness training* (Canton, OH: Professional Reports Corporation), 146.

Form 19

Progress Notes

Date _____

Physician _____

Member's name _____

Weight _____ Date of last program review _____

Medical history changes _____

_____

_____

Exercise prescription _____

_____

_____

Comments _____

_____

_____

Form 20

Incident Report Form

Date of accident _____ Time of accident _____

Member's name _____ Member number _____

Address _____

Home phone _____ Business phone _____

Location of accident _____

Staff attending _____ _____

_____ _____

Witnesses (nonstaff) _____ _____

_____ _____

Details of accident _____

_____

_____

_____

Action taken by staff _____

_____

_____

_____

Staff reporting _____ Date _____

Department head's signature _____ Date _____

Note. The law varies from state to state. No form should be adopted or used by any program without individualized legal advice.

Form 21
Theft Report Form

Date of accident _____ Time of accident _____

Item reported missing _____

Member's name _____ Member number _____

Address _____

Home phone _____ Business phone _____

Location of accident _____

Description of incident _____

_____

_____

_____

Witnesses _____   _____

_____   _____

Reporting by _____ Date and time _____

Action taken _____

_____

_____

_____

Supervisor's signature _____ Date _____

Form 22

Special Event Sign-Up Sheet

Event _____   Location _____

Date(s) _____   Time(s) _____

Staff responsible _____

Member's name	Number	Member phone no.	Paid	Comments	Follow call
1.					
2.					
3.					
4.					
5.					
6.					
7.					
8.					
9.					
10.					
11.					
12.					
13.					
14.					
15.					
16.					
17.					
18.					
19.					
20.					
21.					
22.					
23.					
24.					
25.					
26.					
27.					
28.					
29.					
30.					

Form 23

Appointment Sheet

Time	Name/length	Member number	Phone number	CNL	Date	INT	CONF
8:00							
8:15							
8:30							
8:45							
9:00							
9:15							
9:30							
9:45							
10:00							
10:15							
10:30							
10:45							
11:00							
11:15							
11:30							
11:45							
12:00							
12:15							
12:30							
12:45							
1:00							
1:15							
1:30							
1:45							
2:00							
2:15							
2:30							
2:45							
3:00							
3:15							
3:30							
3:45							
4:00							
4:15							
4:30							
4:45							
5:00							
5:15							
5:30							
5:45							
6:00							
6:15							
6:30							
6:45							
7:00							
7:15							
7:30							
7:45							
8:00							
8:15							
8:30							

DAY _____

_____ / _____

DATE

Therapist _____

Hours

Therapist _____

Hours _____

- Use Pencil
- Mark out 15 minutes before and after the appointment
- **Last appointments:**
  Mon-Thur
      7:30 pm
  Fri   **7:00 pm**
  Sat   **1:00 pm**
- Remind gift certificate and coupon holders to bring them
- Remind clients of cancellation policy and check column that you did remind them

  3-hour notice, or a cancellation fee of $10.00 will be charged

Appointments Confirmed

by _____

at _____

on _____

Form 24

Sample Exercise Card

Sex   M ☐   F ☐   Age _____

Resting heart rate _____   Resting blood pressure _____

History _____

Training pulse _____

Example:

| wt / sets + reps |

Activity	Prescription										
Resting	H.R. ___ ___ /										
	B.P. ___ /										
Warm-up exercises											
1.											
2.											
3.											
4.											
5.											
6.											
7.											
8.											
9.											
10.											
11.											
12.											
13.											
14.											
15.											
16.											
17.											
18.											
19.											

Seat heights

Member name _____

Member number _____

Personal fitness motivator's initials _____

Please see your motivator when finished with your card.

Form 25

Physical Activity Readiness Medical Exam Form (PARmed-X)

The PARmed-X is a physical activity-specific checklist to be used by a physician with patients who have had positive responses to the Physical Activity Readiness Questionnaire (PAR-Q). In addition, the Conveyance/Referral Form in the PARmed-X can be used to convey clearance for physical activity participation, or to make a referral to a medically-supervised exercise program.

Regular physical activity is fun and healthy, and increasingly more people are starting to become more active every day. Being more active is very safe for most people. The PAR-Q by itself provides adequate screening for the majority of people. However, some individuals may require a medical evaluation and specific advice (exercise prescription) due to one or more positive responses to the PAR-Q.

Following the participant's evaluation by a physician, a physical activity plan should be devised in consultation with a physical activity professional (CSEP-Certified Fitness Appraiser). To assist in this, the following instructions are provided:

Page 1: • Sections A, B, C, and D should be completed by the participant BEFORE the examination by the physician. The bottom section is to be completed by the examining physician.

Pages 2 & 3: • A checklist of medical conditions requiring special consideration and management.

This section to be completed by the participant

A PERSONAL INFORMATION:

Name _____

Address _____

_____

Telephone _____

Birthdate _____ Gender _____

Medical No. _____

B PAR-Q: Please indicate the PAR-Q questions to which you answered YES

❑ Q1. Heart condition
❑ Q2. Chest pain during activity
❑ Q3. Chest pain at rest
❑ Q4. Loss of balance, dizziness
❑ Q5. Bone or joint problem
❑ Q6. Blood pressure or heart drugs
❑ Q7. Other reason:

C RISK FACTORS FOR CARDIOVASCULAR DISEASE:
Check all that apply

❑ Less than 30 minutes of moderate physical activity most days of the week.
❑ Currently smoker (tobacco smoking 1 or more times per week).
❑ High blood pressure reported by physician after repeated measurements.
❑ High cholesterol level reported by physician.

❑ Excessive accumulation of fat around waist.
❑ Family history of heart disease.

Please note: *Many of these risk factors are modifiable. Please discuss with your physician.*

D PHYSICAL ACTIVITY INTENTIONS:

What physical activity do you intend to do?

_____

_____

_____

This section to be completed by the examining physician

Physical Exam:

Ht	Wt		BP i)	/
			BP ii)	/

Conditions limiting physical activity:

❑ Cardiovascular ❑ Respiratory ❑ Other
❑ Musculoskeletal ❑ Abdominal

Tests required:

❑ ECG ❑ Exercise test ❑ X-Ray
❑ Blood ❑ Urinalysis ❑ Other

Physical Activity Readiness Conveyance/Referral:
Based upon a current review of health status, I recommend:

❑ No physical activity ❑ Only a medically-supervised exercise program until further medical clearance

❑ Progressive physical activity
  ❑ with avoidance of: _____
  ❑ with inclusion of: _____
  ❑ with Physical Therapy: _____

❑ Unrestricted physical activity —start slowly and build up gradually

Further information:
❑ Attached
❑ To be forwarded
❑ Available on request

Following is a checklist of medical conditions for which a degree of precaution and/or special advice should be considered for those who answered "YES" to one or more questions on the PAR-Q, and people over the age of 69. Conditions are grouped by system. Three categories of precautions are provided. Comments under Advice are general, since details and alternatives require clinical judgement in each individual instance.

	Absolute Contraindications	Relative Contraindications	Special Prescriptive Conditions	ADVICE
	Permanent restriction or temporary restriction until condition is treated, stable, and/or past acute phase.	Highly variable. Value of exercise testing and/or program may exceed risk. Activity may be restricted. Desirable to maximize control of condition. Direct or indirect medical supervision or exercise program may be desirable.	Individualized prescriptive advice generally appropriate: • limitations imposed; and/or • special exercises prescribed. May require medical monitoring and/or initial supervision in exercise program.	
Cardiovascular	❏ aortic aneurysm (dissecting) ❏ aortic stenosis (severe) ❏ congestive heart failure ❏ crescendo angina ❏ myocardial infarction (acute) ❏ myocarditis (active or recent) ❏ pulmonary or systemic embolism—acute ❏ thrombophlebitis ❏ ventricular tachycardia and other dangerous dysrhythmias (e.g., multi-focal ventricular activity)	❏ aortic stenosis (moderate) ❏ subaortic stenosis (severe) ❏ marked cardiac enlargement ❏ supraventricular dysrhythmias (uncontrolled or high rate) ❏ ventricular ectopic activity (repetitive or frequent) ❏ ventricular aneurysm ❏ hypertension—untreated or uncontrolled severe (systemic or pulmonary) ❏ hypertrophic cardiomyopathy ❏ compensated congestive heart failure	❏ aortic (or pulmonary) stenosis—mild angina pectoris and other manifestations of coronary insufficiency (e.g., post-acute infarct) ❏ cyanotic heart disease ❏ shunts (intermittent or fixed) ❏ conduction disturbances • complete AV block • left BBB • Wolff-Parkinson-White syndrome ❏ dysrhythmias—controlled ❏ fixed rate pacemakers	• clinical exercise test may be warranted in selected cases, for specific determination of functional capacity and limitations and precautions (if any). • slow progression of exercise to levels based on test performance and individual tolerance. • consider individual need for initial conditioning program under medical supervision (indirect or direct).
			❏ intermittent claudication	progressive exercise to tolerance
			❏ hypertension: systolic 160-180; diastolic 105+	progressive exercise; care with medications (serum electrolytes; post-exercise syncope; etc.)
Infections	❏ acute infectious disease (regardless of etiology)	❏ subacute/chronic/recurrent infectious diseases (e.g., malaria, others)	❏ chronic infections ❏ HIV	variable as to condition
Metaboli		❏ uncontrolled metabolic disorders (diabetes mellitus, thyrotoxicosis, myxedema)	❏ renal, hepatic & other metabolic insufficiency	variable as to status
			❏ obesity ❏ single kidney	dietary moderation, and initial light exercises with slow progression (walking, swimming, cycling)
Pregnancy		❏ complicated pregnancy (e.g., toxemia, hemorrhage, incompetent cervix, etc.)	❏ advanced pregnancy (late 3rd trimester)	refer to the "PARmed-X for PREGNANCY"

References:

Arraix, G.A., Wigle, D.T., Mao, Y. (1992). Risk Assessment of Physical Activity and Physical Fitness in the Canada Health Survey Follow-Up Study. **J. Clin. Epidemiol. 45:4 419-428.**

Mottola, M., Wolfe, L.A. (1994). Active Living and Pregnancy, In: A. Quinney, L. Gauvin, T. Wall (eds), **Toward Active Living: Proceedings of the International Conference on Physical Activity, Fitness and Health.** Champaign, IL: Human Kinetics.

PAR-Q Validation Report, British Columbia Ministry of Health, 1978.

Thomas, S., Reading, J., Shephard, R.J. (1992). Revision of the Physical Activity Readiness Questionnaire (PAR-Q). **Can. J. Spt. Sci.** 17:4 338-345.

	Special Prescriptive Conditions	**Advice**
Lung	❏ chronic pulmonary disorders	special relaxation and breathing exercises
	❏ obstructive lung disease ❏ asthma	breath control during endurance exercise to tolerance; avoid polluted air
	❏ exercise-induced bronchospasm	avoid hyperventilation during exercise; avoid extremely cold conditions; warm up adequately; utilize appropriate medication
Musculoskeletal	❏ low back conditions (pathological, functional)	avoid or minimize exercise that precipitates or exacerbates (e.g., forced extreme flexion, extension, and violent twisting); correct posture, proper back exercises
	❏ arthritis—acute (infective, rheumatoid; gout)	treatment, plus judicious blend of rest, splinting, and gentle movement
	❏ arthritis—subacute	progressive increase of active exercise therapy
	❏ arthritis—chronic (osteoarthritis and above conditions)	maintenance of mobility and strength; non-weightbearing exercises to minimize joint trauma (e.g., cycling, aquatic activity, etc.)
	❏ orthopaedic	highly variable and individualized
	❏ hernia	minimize straining and isometrics; strengthen abdominal muscles
CNS	❏ convulsive disorder not completely controlled by medication	minimize or avoid exercise in hazardous environments and/or exercising alone (e.g., swimming, mountain climbing, etc.)
	❏ recent concussion	thorough examination if history of two concussions; review for discontinuation of contact sport if three concussions, depending on duration of unconsciousness, retrograde amnesia, persistent headaches, and other objective evidence of cerebral damage
Blood	❏ anemia—severe (< 10 Gm/dl) ❏ electrolyte disturbances	control preferred; exercise as tolerated
Medications	❏ antianginal ❏ antiarrhythmic ❏ antihypertensive ❏ anticonvulsant ❏ beta-blockers ❏ digitalis preparations ❏ diuretics ❏ ganglionic blockers ❏ others	NOTE: consider underlying condition. Potential for: exertional syncope, electrolyte imbalance, bradycardia, dysrhythmias, impaired coordinations and reaction time, heat intolerance. May alter resting and exercise ECG's and exercise test performance.
Other	❏ post-exercise syncope	moderate program
	❏ heat intolerance	prolong cool-down with light activities; avoid exercise in extreme heat
	❏ temporary minor illness	postpone until recovered
	❏ cancer	if potential metastases, test by cycle ergometry, consider non-weight bearing exercises; exercise at lower end of prescriptive range (40-65% of heart rate reserve), depending on condition and recent treatment (radiation, chemotherapy); monitor hemoglobin and lymphocyte counts; add dynamic lifting exercises to strengthen muscles, using machines rather than weights.

* Refer to special publications for elaboration as required.

Form 26

Emergency Procedures Sheet

In the event that an emergency should occur and no medical personnel are present, the following guidelines should be followed:

1. A staff person should identify him or herself as a professional rescuer trained in emergency care. This helps to reassure the victim and bystanders. If the victim is conscious, legally we must ask permission to assist the victim. (The law assumes that an unconscious person would give consent.) A senior staff person should stay with the individual at all times. He or she should attempt to reassure the person and protect the individual from personal bodily harm. Senior staff person will assume control of the situation and issue further orders as needed.

2. A second staff member will call 911 and give the following information:

   A. Phone number of location

   B. Title of location (building name, address, specific suite or room number)

   C. Site-specific entrance instructions for ambulance driver

   D. Brief description of the problem. If it is a definite cardiac event (i.e., respiratory arrest) and CPR is in progress, an Advanced Life Support unit will be sent. If it is nonlife-threatening (i.e., seizures), a Basic Life Support unit will be sent.

   E. After 911 has been called, a staff member will notify building security (list phone #: _____), put elevator on hold (if applicable), and wait in the lobby to meet the ambulance at the main entrance to escort them to the emergency.

3. The individual should be monitored at all times. This will include:

   A. Checking heart rate, noting the regularity and strength of each heart beat.

   B. Monitoring and recording blood pressure.

   C. Observing skin color and breathing pattern.

   D. Maintaining open airway.

   E. Establishing unresponsiveness and initiating CPR when appropriate.

   F. Before the individual is transported (if unconscious), give the EMTs as much information as possible regarding individual's name, age, medical considerations (folder, if possible), and home phone emergency numbers. The attending physician and the hospital will make the call to the family.

4. Once the individual is transported, the senior staff person in charge should:

   A. Notify the individual's work place so that the employer can decide how to handle the family.

   B. Assume responsibility for personal belongings and valuables. Please remember that it is important to respect the individual's privacy. Be as brief as possible when disclosing the information pertinent to the event.

   C. Fill out an accident report and file one copy in the member's folder and one copy with the Center Director.

Form 27

Health Questionnaire

Name _____ Date _____

Address _____

Gender _____ Birthday _____ E-mail _____

Telephone (W) _____ Telephone (H) _____

Regular physical activity is fun and healthy and for most people safe. However, some individuals may have health-related risks that might require them to check with their physician prior to starting an exercise program. To help determine if there is a need for you to see your physician before starting an exercise program, please read the following questions and answer carefully.

All information will be kept in the strictest confidentiality. In addition to the health history questions, we have also listed several questions pertaining to your interests and goals for participating in an exercise/physical activity program.

I. PHYSICAL ACTIVITY SCREENING QUESTIONS

Yes   No

☐ ☐ 1. Has your physician ever told you that you have a heart condition?

☐ ☐ 2. Do you experience pain in your chest when you are physically active?

☐ ☐ 3. In the past month, have you experienced chest pain when not performing physical activity?

☐ ☐ 4. Do you lose balance because of dizziness or do you ever lose consciousness?

☐ ☐ 5. Do you have a bone or joint problem that could be aggravated by a change in your level of physical activity?

☐ ☐ 6. Is your physician currently prescribing medications for your blood pressure or heart condition?

☐ ☐ 7. Do you know of any other reason why you should not participate in a program of physical activity?

If you answered yes to any of the above questions, it is recommended that you consult with your physician via phone or in person before having a fitness test or participating in a physical activity program.

II. GENERAL HEALTH HISTORY QUESTIONS

Yes   No

☐ ☐ 1. Have you ever experienced a stroke?

☐ ☐ 2. Do you have diabetes? If yes, are you currently taking any medications or receiving other treatment related to the diabetes? _____

☐ ☐ 3. Do you have asthma or another respiratory condition that causes difficulty with breathing? If yes, please describe. _____

☐ ☐ 4. Do you have any orthopedic conditions that would restrict you in performing physical activity? If yes, please describe. _____

☐ ☐ 5. Have you ever been told by a physician that you have one of the following? (check applicable boxes) ☐ High blood pressure   ☐ Elevated blood lipids, including cholesterol

☐ ☐ 6. Do you currently smoke?

☐ ☐ 7. Have you experienced within the past 6 months back pain or discomfort that prevented you from carrying out normal daily activities?

☐ ☐ 8. Are you pregnant?

☐ ☐ 9. Do you currently exercise less than one hour per week? If you answered no, please describe your activities: _____

☐ ☐ 10. Are you currently taking any medications that might impact your ability to safely perform physical activity?

I. ACTIVITY RELEASE AGREEMENT: ADULT

I am voluntarily participating in an athletic or physical activity at ("the club") with full knowledge and understanding and appreciation of the risks of injury inherent in any physical exercise, massage or therapy program, physical activity, or athletic activity and expressly assume all risks of injury and even death, which could occur by reason of my participation. I release the club from any liability and agree not to sue the club with respect to any cause of action for bodily injury, property damage, or death occurring to me as a result of my participation in the activity.

I understand that all personal property brought to the club is brought at my sole risk as to its theft, damage, or loss.

Participant   Witness
Signature _____   Signature _____

Date _____   Date _____

Printed name _____   Printed name _____

II. FOR MEMBERSHIP/ATHLETIC USE ONLY

Category 1 _____   Category 2 _____   Category 3 _____

Form 28

Coronary Risk Factor Identification Form

Member name _____ Member # _____ Date _____

Place a check next to any lines below that apply to the member.

1. _____ **Age:** (Circle)   Men>45   Women >55

2. _____ **Family history:** MI or sudden death before 55 years of age for father or other first degree male relative

   MI or sudden death before 65 years of age for mother or other first degree female relative

3. _____ **Cigarette smoker:** (Current)

4. _____ **Hypercholesterolemia:** Blood cholesterol > 200 mg/dl

5. _____ **Hypertension:** Blood pressure > 140/90 mm Hg or on hypertensive meds.

6. _____ **Diabetes mellitus:** Classified with disease as follows:

   ☐ NIDDM > 35 years or older.

   ☐ IDDM > older than 30 or having IDDM for 15 years minimum.

7. _____ **Sedentary lifestyle:** Physical inactivity.

_____ **Apparently healthy:**
Asymptomatic and apparently healthy with no more than one major coronary risk factor.

Risk factors: _____

_____

_____

_____ **Increased risk:**
An individual who has signs or symptoms suggestive of possible cardiopulmonary or metabolic disease and/or two or more major coronary risk factors.

Risk factors: _____

_____

_____

Physician's note required   Date contacted: _____

_____ **Known disease:**
An individual with known cardiac, pulmonary, or metabolic disease.

Risk factors: _____

_____

_____

Physician's note required   Date contacted: _____

Form 29

Fitness Testing Form

Name _____ Member # _____ Gender _____ Age _____

		INITIAL	30 DAY	60 DAY
DATE				
RESTING HR				
Resting BP				
	Systolic			
	Diastolic			
Circumferences				
	Biceps			
	Chest			
	Waist			
	Hip			
	Thigh			
Skinfolds				
	Pectoral (M)			
	Abdominal (M)			
	Thigh (F/M)			
	Tricep (F)			
	Suprailliac			
	Sum			
	% body fat			
3-minute step test				
	HR			
	Fitness level			
Push-ups				
Flexibility				
	Sit and reach			
Height				
Weight				

Form 30

Medical Clearance Form

Information requested for _____

Physician's name _____

Telephone number _____

Please sign the statement that reflects your wishes:

1. _____ I concur with my patient's participation if he/she restricts activities to those that are moderate.

2. _____ I do not concur with my patient's participation in this program. (If checked, the individual will not be accepted.)

3. _____ Other: _____

_____

Return form to: _____

Form 31

Exercise Contract

Member name _____

Member contact no. (W) _____ (H) _____ (C) _____

Fitness motivator _____

Motivator contact no. (W) _____ (H) _____ (C) _____

Goals and Objectives

My main exercise goal is to _____

To achieve my main goal, I need to do the following:

a. 30-day goal _____
_____

b. 60-day goal _____
_____

c. 90-day goal _____
_____

d. 6-month goal _____
_____

I commit to do the following:

1. Cardiovascular _____
_____

2. Strength training _____
_____

3. Nutrition _____
_____

4. Flexibility _____
_____

What barriers do you expect might arise to prevent you from achieving your goals and how can we assist in overcoming them?

Exercise Contract Overview

1. When establishing this contract with a Member, be certain to set SMART goals *(Specific, Measurable, Achievable, Realistic, and Timed).*

2. To help achieve the desired results, use the following options as incentives to keep the Member motivated:

   a. If not yet committed to an exercise program. Additional training sessions, setting them up with an exercise "buddy" in the same exercise situation, discounts for club services such as massage, lessons, classes, etc., educational materials on benefits of exercise, group training sessions, and incentives or rewards.

   b. If already participating in a program but just recently started. The focus is on preventing lapses (short breaks from exercise) and relapses (long periods of inactivity). Use buddy programs and group training options for social support. Additional complimentary training and incentives rewards work well also.

3. The support you provide as the motivator is critical to the success.

Form 32

Health, Fitness, and Racquet Sports Club Incident Report

(Complete for all incidents and report immediately—please print)

D A T E	Month Day Year Time of Accident A.M. P.M.	Club member ☐ Yes ☐ No	Club name Club location

I N J U R E D P E R S O N	First name (M.I.) Last name Age	Hospital or first aid squad notified ☐ Yes ☐ No Name:
		Time of initial call:
	Number and street	Times of follow-up calls: 1. 3. 2. 4.
		Time of arrival:
	City State Zip	Time of departure:
		Taken to hospital?
	Business phone Home phone	Name of first aid attendant:

DESCRIPTION OF ACCIDENT:

CHECK ITEMS THAT APPLY TO INJURED PERSON:

Bleeding injury: ☐ Yes ☐ No   Other visible injury: ☐ Yes ☐ No

No visible injury, but complaint of pain: ☐ Yes ☐ No

If eye injury, wearing eyeguards? ☐ Yes ☐ No

DESCRIBE EXACT INJURY SUSTAINED:	**DESCRIBE FIRST AID ADMINISTERED BY CLUB:**

FIRST WITNESS	**SECOND WITNESS**
First name (M.I.) Last name	First name (M.I.) Last name
Number and street	Number and street
City State Zip	City State Zip
Business phone Home phone	Business phone Home phone
DESCRIPTION OF ACCIDENT BY WITNESS	**DESCRIPTION OF ACCIDENT BY WITNESS**
Signature:	Signature:

| HEALTH, FITNESS & RACQUET SPORTS CLUB INCIDENT REPORT |
| [continued] |

Name of club personnel who inspected the scene: _____

Position _____

Date of inspection _____

Conditions found: _____

_____

_____

_____

Action taken, if practical, to avoid recurrence: _____

_____

DESCRIPTION OF PLACE OF ACCIDENT

☐ Interior ☐ Exterior ☐ Walking area ☐ Playing surface ☐ Locker room

☐ Physical fitness room ☐ Other: _____

Conditions: ☐ Dry ☐ Wet ☐ Smooth ☐ Even surface ☐ Slippery

Foreign substance? ☐ Yes ☐ No If "YES", description: _____

If injury took place outside club building, check appropriate items:

Weather condition: ☐ Dry ☐ Rain ☐ Snow ☐ Ice ☐ Day ☐ Night Lighting conditions: _____

IMPORTANT: If injury took place on a court, provide name, address, and telephone number of those individuals who used or rented the court during the prior hour.

_____

_____

ADDITIONAL COMMENTS

_____

_____

Did police investigate? Name and rank of officer: _____ Department: _____ Phone number _____

☐ Yes ☐ No

Submitted by (signature): _____ Telephone: _____ Date / Time _____

This information is for reporting purposes only. The information provided is the responsibility of the insured and/or club.

Form 33

Housekeeping Checklist—Fitness Equipment Room

Note: Follow manufacturer's recommendation for maintaining belts, rods, bearings, chains, gears, and upholstered surfaces of exercise equipment.

DAILY

_____ Remove trash for disposal and replace liners

_____ Dust all horizontal surfaces

_____ Spot-clean mirrors and glass

_____ Spot-clean doors, door handles, light switches, trash containers, etc.

_____ Spot-clean walls

_____ Clean and disinfect all benches and equipment

_____ Polish vinyl pad surfaces with furniture polish

_____ Vacuum carpets

_____ Remove spots and stains from carpet

_____ Spray odor counteractant

BIMONTHLY

_____ Completely clean mirrors, rubber floor, equipment, benches, etc.

_____ Clean HVAC vents

_____ Clean light fixtures

_____ Move all equipment and clean underneath

QUARTERLY

_____ Bonnet-clean carpets

YEARLY

_____ Extraction-clean carpets

_____ Wash all walls

MAINTENANCE
Report any repairs required

_____

_____

_____

_____

_____

PEST CONTROL
Report any evidence of insects or rodents

_____

_____

_____

_____

_____

1. DAILY MAINTENANCE

A. Trash removal

Purpose: Provide a clean, well-maintained area for all members using the facility

Frequency: Daily or more frequently depending on the amount of traffic

Techniques: Remove trash and replace liners

B. Cleaning and disinfecting of workout equipment room surfaces

Purpose: Provide clean, sanitary, odor-free area for all members

Frequency: Daily or more frequently depending on the amount of traffic and soil levels

Techniques: Vacuum carpet, remove carpet spots and stains, clean and disinfect benches and equipment, spot-clean any mirror surfaces, door handles, doors, light switches, and walls

2. BIMONTHLY MAINTENANCE: FULL WET CLEANING OF ALL SURFACES

Purpose: To completely clean all room surfaces including mirrors, vents, light fixtures, rubber floor, equipment, benches, doors, etc.

Frequency: Every two weeks

Technique: Completely clean any mirrors, vents, light fixtures, rubber floor, equipment, benches, doors, etc.

3. BIMONTHLY MAINTENANCE: MOVE ALL EQUIPMENT AND CLEAN UNDERNEATH

Purpose: To completely clean all room surfaces

Frequency: Every two weeks

Technique: Move all equipment and clean underneath, vacuum or dust mop and damp mop as required

4. QUARTERLY MAINTENANCE: CARPET CLEANING

Purpose: To clean traffic lanes of carpet and maintain a high level of appearance

Frequency: Every three months

Technique: Bonnet-clean carpets

5. YEARLY MAINTENANCE: CARPET CLEANING AND WALL WASHING

Purpose: Provide a high level of appearance and odor free environment

Frequency: Yearly

Technique: Clean carpets and wash walls

Form 34

Housekeeping Checklist—Locker Room

Date _____

Housekeeper _____

DAILY

_____ Remove trash for disposal and replace liners

_____ Refill paper, hand soap, shampoo, conditioner dispensers, etc.

_____ Dust and polish all furniture and touch-up other wood surfaces

_____ Dust all horizontal surfaces

_____ Spot-clean mirrors and glass

_____ Spot-clean doors, door handles, light switches, trash containers, etc.

_____ Spot-clean walls

_____ Spot-clean lockers

_____ Clean and disinfect sinks, commodes, urinals, etc.

_____ Clean and disinfect showers, sauna, steam room, and whirlpool

_____ Vacuum carpets

_____ Remove spots and stains from carpet

_____ Dust mop or sweep hard surface floors

_____ Wet mop and disinfect hard surface floors

_____ Spray odor counteractant

BIMONTHLY

_____ Clean mirrors, glass, and locker surfaces completely

_____ Clean hard surface floors by scrubbing with deck brush or machine

_____ Clean and disinfect showers, steam room, sauna, and whirlpool

_____ Clean HVAC vents

_____ Clean light fixtures

MONTHLY

_____ Refill air freshener dispensers

QUARTERLY

_____ Bonnet-clean carpets

YEARLY

_____ Extraction-clean carpets

_____ Wash all walls

MAINTENANCE
Report any repairs required

_____

_____

_____

_____

PEST CONTROL
Report any evidence of insects or rodents

_____

_____

_____

_____

OVERVIEW

1. Daily Maintenance

   A. Trash removal, refilling paper supplies and hand soap and other dispensers

   Purpose: Provide a well-maintained locker room for all members using the facility

   Frequency: Daily or more frequently depending on the amount of traffic

   Techniques: Refill all toilet paper, paper towel, seat covers, and liquid hand soap dispensers

   B. Cleaning and disinfecting of locker room surfaces

   Purpose: Provide clean, sanitary, odor-free locker room area for all members

   Frequency: Daily or more frequently depending on the amount of traffic and soil levels

   Techniques: Wet cleaning and disinfecting of all surfaces, including lockers, fixtures, showers, walls, partitions, steam room, sauna, whirlpool, floors, and wood surface touch-up
   Spot mop cleaning and disinfecting should be performed on spills when they occur.

2. Bimonthly Maintenance: Full Wet Cleaning and Disinfecting

   Purpose: To completely clean and disinfect all locker room surfaces including lockers, fixtures, showers, walls, partitions, steam room, sauna, whirlpool, and doors; clean and polish furniture and other wood surfaces

   Frequency: Every two weeks

   Technique: Completely clean and disinfect fixtures, walls, floors, vents, and light fixtures

3. Quarterly Maintenance: Carpet Cleaning

   Purpose: To clean traffic lanes of carpet and maintain a high level of appearance

   Frequency: Every three months

   Technique: Bonnet-clean carpets

4. Yearly Maintenance: Carpet Extraction Cleaning and Wall Washing

   Purpose: Provide a high level of appearance and odor free environment

   Frequency: Yearly

   Technique: Extraction-clean carpets and wash walls

Accessible Sports Facilities

A Summary of Accessibility Guidelines for Recreational Facilities

INTRODUCTION

The Americans with Disabilities Act (ADA) is a comprehensive civil rights law that prohibits discrimination on the basis of disability. The ADA requires that newly constructed and altered state and local government facilities, places of public accommodation, and commercial facilities be readily accessible to, and usable by, individuals with disabilities. The ADA Accessibility Guidelines (ADAAG) is the standard applied to buildings and facilities. Recreational facilities, including sports facilities, are among the facilities required to comply with the ADA.

The Access Board issued accessibility guidelines for newly constructed and altered recreation facilities in 2002. The recreation facility guidelines are a supplement to ADAAG. As a supplement, they must be used in conjunction with ADAAG. References to ADAAG are mentioned throughout this summary. Copis of ADAAG and the recreation facility accessibility guidelines can be obtained through the Board's Web site at www.access-board.gov or by calling 1-800-872-2253 or 1-800-993-2822 (TTY). Once these guidelines are adopted by the Department of Justice (DOJ), all newly designed, constructed, and altered recreation facilities coveredy by the ADA will be required to comply.

Material in appendix C appears courtesy of United States Access Board.

The recreation facility guidelines cover the following facilities and elements:

- Amusement rides
- Boating facilities
- Bowling lanes
- Exercise equipment
- Fishing piers and platforms
- Golf courses
- Miniature golf courses
- Shooting facilities
- Swimming pools, wading pools, and spas

This guide is intended to help designers and operators in using the accessibility guidelines for sports facilities. These guidelines establish minimum accessibility requirements for newly designed or newly constructed and altered sports facilities. This guide is not a collection of sports facility designs. Rather, it provides specifications for elements within a sports facility to create a general level of usability for individuals with disabilities. Emphasis is placed on ensuring that individuals with disabilities are generally able to access the sports facility and use a variety of elements.

Designers and operators are encouraged to exceed the guidelines where possible to provide increased accessibility and opportunities. Incorporating accessibility into the design of a sports facility should begin early in the planning process with careful consideration of accessible routes.

The recreation facility guidelines were developed with significant public participation. In 1993, the Access Board established an advisory committee of 27 members to recommend accessibility guidelines for recreation facilities. The Recreation Access Advisory Committee represented the following groups and associations:

- American Ski Federation
- American Society for Testing and Materials (Public Playground Safety Committee)
- American Society of Landscape Architects
- Beneficial Designs
- City and County of San Francisco, California, Department of Public Works
- Disabled American Veterans
- Environmental Access
- Gold Course Superintendents Association of America
- Hawaii Disability and Communication Access Board
- International Association of Amusement Parks and Attractions
- Katherine McGuinness and Associates
- Lehman, Smith, and Wiseman Associates
- Michigan Department of Natural Resources
- National Council on Independent Living
- National Park Service
- National Recreation and Park Association
- New Jersey Department of Community Affairs
- Outdoor Amusement Business Association
- Paralyzed Veterans of America
- Professional Golfer's Association
- Self Help for Hard of Hearing People
- States Organization for Boating Access
- Universal Studios
- U.S. Army Corps of Engineers
- U.S. Forest Service
- YMCA of the USA
- Walt Disney Imagineering

The public was given an opportunity to comment on the recommended accessibility guidelines, and the Access Board made changes to the recommended guidelines based on the public comments. A notice of proposed rulemaking (NPRM) was published in the Federal Register in July 1999, followed by a five-month public comment period. Further input from the public was sought in July 2000 when the Access Board published a draft final rule soliciting comment. A final rule was published in September 2002.

"Whenever a door is closed to anyone because of a disability, we must work to open it. . . . Whenever any barrier stands between you and the full rights and dignity of citizenship, we must work to remove it, in the name of simple decency and justice. The promise of the ADA . . . has enabled people with disabilities to enjoy much greater access to a wide range of affordable travel, recreational opportunities, and life-enriching services."

—President George W. Bush,
New Freedom Initiative,
February 1, 2001

SPORTS FACILITIES

The recreation facility guidelines described in this guide focus on the accessible features of unique sports-related elements in newly designed or newly constructed and altered facilities. Other provisions contained in ADAAG address elements commonly found within a sports facility, such as accessible vehicle parking spaces, exterior accessible routes, doors, assembly sections, and toilet and bathing facilities. ADAAG addresses only the built environment (structures and grounds). The guidelines do not address operational issues. Questions regarding operational issues should be directed to the Department of Justice, 1-800-514-0301 or 1-800-514-0383 (TTY).

Facilities and elements covered include:

- Areas of indoor and outdoor sports activity, including court sports (such as tennis, volleyball, and racquetball), field sports (such as softball, football, lacrosse, baseball, and soccer), and other sports (such as gymnastics and wrestling)
- Dressing, fitting, and locker rooms
- Team or player seating areas
- Exercise equipment and machines

- Saunas and steam rooms
- Animal containment areas for public use such as petting zoos and passageways along animal pens at fairs
- Bowling lanes
- Shooting facilities

These recreation facility guidelines do not apply to:

- Raised structures used for refereeing, judging, or scoring a sport
- Animal containment areas not for public use
- Raised boxing rings and wrestling rings
- Water slides (as long as an accessible route is provided to the base)

ACCESSIBLE ROUTES

Accessible routes are continuous, unobstructed paths connecting all accessible elements and spaces of a building or facility. The accessible route must comply with ADAAG provisions for the location,

width (minimum of 36 inches), passing space, head room, surface, slope (maximum of 1:12 or 8.33 percent), changes in level, doors, egress, and areas of rescue assistance, unless otherwise modified by specific provisions outlined in this guide. Facilities must provide accessible routes connecting all accessible elements and spaces within areas of indoor or outdoor sports activities. If not all elements need to be accessible, only those that are accessible must be connected with an accessible route.

The guidelines apply to "fixed" facilities and elements. They do not cover equipment that is frequently moved. For example, a wrestling mat or badminton net may be portable and moved regularly.

Court Sports

Where courts are provided, an accessible route must connect each court. Accessible routes must comply with all ADAAG requirements, such as width and changes in level or surface, and must directly connect both sides of the court. Players must not be required to traverse through another court to get to the other side of their court. This is especially critical in sports like tennis, in which changing sides of the

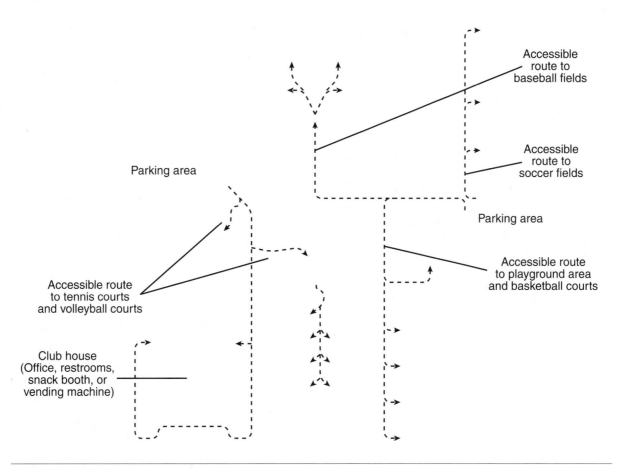

Accessible route connecting various elements of a multiuse facility.

Exit to parking

Accessible route connecting court sports.

court is part of the game. No additional accessibility guidelines apply once on the court.

Areas of Sport Activities

An "area of sport activity" is a broad term intended to cover a diverse number of indoor and outdoor sports fields and areas. This includes, but is not limited to: basketball courts, baseball fields, running tracks, soccer fields, and skating rinks.

The "area of sport activity" is "that portion of a room or space where the play or practice of a sport occurs." For example, football fields are defined by boundary lines. In addition, a safety border is provided around the field. Players may temporarily be in the space between the boundary lines and the safety border when they are pushed out of bounds or momentum carries them forward when receiving a pass. So in football, that space is used as part of the game and is included in the area of sport activity.

Accessible routes must connect each area of sport activity. Areas of sport activities must comply with all ADAAG requirements, except that they are exempt from the requirement that surfaces must be stable, firm, and slip resistant, and from the restrictions on carpets, grating, and changes in level. They are also exempt from restrictions on protruding objects. These provisions are not required inside of the area of sport activity since they may affect the fundamental nature of the sport or activity. For example, an accessible route is required to connect to the boundary of a soccer field, but there is no requirement to change the surface of a field to an accessible surface.

Where light fixtures or gates are provided as part of a court sport or other area of sport activity, they must comply with ADAAG provisions for controls and operating mechanisms, and for gates and doors.

Animal Containment Areas

If the public has access to an animal containment area, accessible routes must connect to each animal containment area. Examples may include petting zoos, petting farms, public pathways for viewing livestock display tents, or other areas where the public has access to animals. These areas must comply with all ADAAG requirements, except the requirements that surfaces be stable, firm, and slip resistant and the restrictions on changes in level since some surfaces need to be absorbent. Accessibility is not required in areas that are for animal handlers and not for public use.

DRESSING, FITTING, OR LOCKER ROOMS

When provided, dressing, fitting, or locker rooms must be accessible and comply with all ADAAG provisions. If they are in a cluster, 5 percent, or at least one, must be accessible. There must be an accessible route through the door and to all elements required to be accessible in the room. Operating mechanisms provided on accessible lockers must also meet ADAAG provisions for their operation and height.

LOCKERS

If lockers are provided, at least 5 percent, but not less than one of each type (full, half, quarter, etc.), must be accessible. Accessible benches should be located adjacent to the accessible lockers.

BENCHES

Accessible benches are required in dressing, fitting, and locker rooms, and where seating is provided in saunas and steam rooms. Benches must have a clear floor space positioned to allow persons using wheelchairs or other mobility devices to approach parallel to the short end of a bench seat. In saunas and steam rooms, this floor space may be obstructed by readily removable seats.

Benches must have seats that are a minimum of 20 inches to a maximum of 24 inches in depth and 42 inches minimum in length. The seat height should be a minimum of 17 inches to a maximum

Accessible lockers.

Accessible bench.

Accessible bench against a wall.

of 19 inches above the finished floor. If the bench is not located next to a wall, the bench must have back support that is 42 inches minimum in length and extends from a point 2 inches maximum above the seat to a point 18 inches minimum above the bench. Benches must be strong enough to withstand a vertical or horizontal force of 250 pounds applied at any point on the seat, fastener, mounting device, or supporting structure. The provisions for benches are not intended to apply to park benches or other benches used for sitting or resting.

If benches are located in wet areas, the surface must be slip-resistant and designed not to accumulate water.

TEAM PLAYER SEATING AREAS

Where provided, fixed team or player seating areas must contain the number of wheelchair spaces and companion seats required by ADAAG (based on the number of seats provided), but not less than one space. One option is to provide a clear space

Accessible team player seating area.

adjacent to a fixed bench, with the bench serving as companion seating. If designers and operators are designing a field or court that will serve a variety of wheelchair sports, exceeding the minimum requirements will better accommodate participants.

Wheelchair spaces in the team player seating areas are exempt from the requirements related to admission price and line of sight choices in assembly areas. It is recommended that ramps be used wherever possible for accessible routes connecting team or player seating areas and areas of sport activity. However, a platform lift may be used as part of an accessible route to team player seating areas.

SAUNAS AND STEAM ROOMS

If saunas or steam rooms are in a cluster, at least 5 percent, but not less than one of each type, must be accessible. The wheelchair turning space in the sauna or steam room must comply with ADAAG, except that it can be obstructed by readily removable seats. If seating is provided, at least one bench must be accessible. Doors cannot swing into any part of the clear floor or ground space required for benches.

EXERCISE EQUIPMENT AND MACHINES

At least one of each type of exercise equipment or machine must have clear floor space of at least 30 by 48 inches and be served by an accessible route. If the clear space is enclosed on three sides (e.g., by walls or the equipment itself), the clear space must be at least 36 by 48 inches.

Most strength training equipment and machines would be considered different types. For example, a bench press machine is different from a biceps curl machine. If operators provide both a biceps curl machine and free weights, both must meet the guidelines in this section even though both can be used to strengthen biceps. Likewise, cardiovascular exercise machines, such as stationary bicycles, rowing machines, stair climbers, and treadmills, are all different types of machines. If the only difference in pieces of equipment provided is that they have different manufacturers, but are the same type, only one must comply.

Clear floor space must be positioned to allow a person to transfer from a wheelchair or to use the equipment while seated in a wheelchair. For example, to make a shoulder press accessible, the clear floor space should be next to the seat. But the clear floor space for a bench press designed for use by a person using a wheelchair would be centered on the operating mechanisms. Clear floor space for more than one piece of equipment may overlap. For example, where different types of exercise equipment and machines are located next to other pieces of equipment, the clear space may be shared. (See figure "Clear space requirements around exercise equipment" on page 155.)

Clear space requirements around exercise equipment.

The exercise equipment and machines themselves do not need to comply with the ADAAG requirements regarding controls and operating mechanisms.

Designers and operators are encouraged to select exercise equipment that provides fitness opportunities for persons with lower body extremity disabilities.

SHOOTING FACILITIES

If facilities provide fixed firing positions, at least 5 percent, but not less than one of each type of fixed firing position, must be served by an accessible route. Fixed firing positions, must have a 60-inch diameter space with slopes not steeper than 1:48 so a wheelchair user can turn around and have a level place from which to shoot.

Types of different firing positions include positions with different admission prices, positions with or without weather covering or lighting, and positions that support different shooting events (e.g., muzzle loading rifle, small bore rifle, high power rifle, bull's eye pistol, action pistol, silhouette, trap, skeet, and archery).

BOWLING LANES

At least 5 percent, but not less than one, of each type of bowling lane must be accessible. (See page 156.) Unlike other areas of sport activity, only those team or player seating areas that serve accessible lanes must be connected with an accessible route and comply with seating requirements. Spectator seating in bowling facilities is addressed in ADAAG and will require wheelchair spaces, companion seating, and designated aisle seats.

Accessible route connecting accessible bowling lanes and team player areas.

MORE INFORMATION

You can obtain copies of the recreation facility guidelines, which include sports facilities, and further technical assistance from the U.S. Access Board at www.access-board.gov, 1-800-872-2253, or 1-800-993-2822 (TTY).

Accessible Swimming Pools and Spas

A Summary of Accessibility Guidelines for Recreation Facilities

INTRODUCTION

The Americans with Disabilities Act (ADA) is a comprehensive civil rights law that prohibits discrimination on the basis of disability. The ADA requires that newly constructed and altered state and local government facilities, places of public accommodation, and commercial facilities be readily accessible to, and usable by, individuals with disabilities. The ADA Accessibility Guidelines (ADAAG) is the standard applied to buildings and facilities. Recreational facilities, including swimming pools, wading pools, and spas, are among the facilities required to comply with the ADA.

The Access Board issued accessibility guidelines for newly constructed and altered recreation facilities in 2002. The recreation facility guidelines are a supplement to ADAAG. As a supplement, they must be used in conjunction with ADAAG. References to ADAAG are mentioned throughout this summary. Copies of ADAAG and the recreation facility accessibility guidelines can be obtained through the Board's Web site at www.access-board.gov or by calling 1-800-872-2253 or 1-800-993-2822 (TTY).

Once these guidelines are adopted by the Department of Justice (DOJ), all newly designed,

constructed, and altered recreation facilities covered by the ADA will be required to comply.

The recreation facility guidelines cover the following facilities and elements:

- Amusement rides
- Boating facilities
- Bowling lanes
- Exercise equipment
- Fishing piers and platforms
- Golf courses
- Miniature golf courses
- Shooting facilities
- Swimming pools, wading pools, and spas

This guide is intended to help designers and operators in using the accessibility guidelines for swimming pools, wading pools, and spas. These guidelines establish minimum accessibility requirements for newly designed or newly constructed and altered swimming pools, wading pools, and spas. This guide is not a collection of swimming pool or spa designs. Rather, it provides specifications for elements within a swimming pool or spa to create a general level of usability for individuals with disabilities. Emphasis is placed on ensuring that individuals with disabilities are generally able to access swimming pools and spas and use a variety of elements. Designers and operators are encouraged to exceed the guidelines where possible to provide increased accessibility and opportunities. Incorporating accessibility into the design of a swimming pool or spa should begin early in the planning process with careful consideration to the accessible routes and means of entry into the water.

The recreation facility guidelines were developed with significant public participation. In 1993, the Access Board established an advisory committee of 27 members to recommend accessibility guidelines for recreation facilities. The Recreation Access Advisory Committee represented the following groups and associations:

- American Ski Federation
- American Society for Testing and Materials (Public Playground Safety Committee)
- American Society of Landscape Architects
- Beneficial Designs
- City and County of San Francisco, California, Department of Public Works
- Disabled American Veterans
- Environmental Access
- Golf Course Superintendents Association of America
- Hawaii Disability and Communication Access Board
- International Association of Amusement Parks and Attractions
- Katherine McGuinness and Associates
- Lehman, Smith, and Wiseman Associates
- Michigan Department of Natural Resources
- National Council on Independent Living
- National Park Service
- National Recreation and Park Association
- New Jersey Department of Community Affairs
- Outdoor Amusement Business Association
- Paralyzed Veterans of America
- Professional Golfer Association
- Self Help for Hard of Hearing People
- States Organization for Boating Access
- Universal Studios
- U.S. Army Corps of Engineers
- U.S. Forest Service
- Y.M.C.A. of the U.S.A.
- Walt Disney Imagineering

The public was given an opportunity to comment on the recommended accessibility guidelines, and the Access Board made changes to the recommended guidelines based on the public comments. A notice of proposed rulemaking (NPRM) was published in the Federal Register in July 1999, followed by a five-month public comment period. Further input from the public was sought in July 2000 when the Access Board published a draft final rule soliciting comment. A final rule was published in September 2002.

> *"Whenever a door is closed to anyone because of a disability, we must work to open it. . . . Whenever any barrier stands between you and the full rights and dignity of citizenship, we must work to remove it, in the name of simple decency and justice. The promise of the ADA . . . has enabled people with disabilities to enjoy much greater access to a wide range of affordable travel, recreational opportunities, and life-enriching services."*
>
> —*President George W. Bush,*
> *New Freedom Initiative,*
> *February 1, 2001*

SWIMMING POOLS AND SPAS

The guidelines described in this guide focus on newly designed or newly constructed and altered swimming pools, wading pools, aquatic recreation facilities, and spas. Other provisions contained in ADAAG address elements commonly found at a swimming facility, such as accessible vehicle parking spaces, exterior accessible routes, and toilet and bathing facilities. ADAAG addresses only the built environment (structures and grounds); the guidelines do not address operational issues. Questions regarding operational issues should be directed to the Department of Justice, 1-800-514-0301 or 1-800-514-0383 (TTY).

ACCESSIBLE ROUTES

Accessible routes are continuous, unobstructed paths connecting all accessible elements and spaces of a building or facility. Accessible route requirements in ADAAG address width (minimum of 36 inches), passing space, head room, surface, slope (maximum of 1:12 or 8.33 percent), changes in level,

Accessible route connecting elements within a multiuse swimming pool facility.

Permitted Means of Pool Access

Pool type	Sloped entry	Lift	Transfer walls	Transfer systems	Stairs
Swimming (less than 300 linear feet of pool wall)	✓	✓			
Swimming (300 or more linear feet of pool wall)—two means of entry required	✓*	✓*	✓	✓	✓
Wave action, leisure river, and other pools where user entry is limited to one area	✓	✓		✓	
Wading pools	✓				
Spas		✓	✓	✓	

*Primary means must be by sloped entry or lift, secondary means can be any of the permitted types.

doors, egress, and areas of rescue assistance, unless modified by specific provisions outlined in this guide. An accessible route is required to provide access to the swimming areas and all the supporting amenities. An accessible route is not required to serve raised diving boards, platforms, or water slides.

TYPES OF FACILITIES AND REQUIRED MEANS OF ENTRY INTO THE WATER

Swimming Pools

Large pools must have a minimum of two accessible means of entry. A large pool is defined as any pool with over 300 linear feet of pool wall. Pool walls at diving areas and in areas where swimmers cannot enter because of landscaping or adjacent structures are still counted as part of the pool's total linear feet.

The primary means of entry must be either a sloped entry into the water or a pool lift that is capable of being independently operated by a person with a disability. The secondary means of entry could be a pool lift, sloped entry, transfer wall, transfer system, or pool stairs. It is recommended that where two means of entry are provided, they be different types and be situated on different pool walls.

Pools with less than 300 linear feet of pool wall are only required to provide one accessible means of entry, which must be either a pool lift or sloped entry.

Aquatic Recreation Facilities

Wave action pools, leisure rivers, sand bottom pools, and other pools where access to the water is limited to one area and where everyone gets in and out at the same place, must provide at least one accessible means of entry, no matter how many linear feet of pool wall is provided. The accessible means of entry can be either a pool lift, sloped entry, or transfer system.

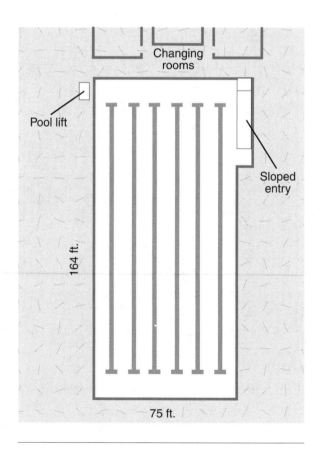

Two means of access required in larger pool.

Zero-grade sloped entry into wave-action pool.

Catch Pools

A catch pool is a body of water where water slide flumes drop users into the water. An accessible means of entry or exit is not required into the catch pool. However, an accessible route must connect to the edge of the catch pool.

Wading Pools

A wading pool is a pool designed for shallow depth and is used for wading. Each wading pool must provide at least one sloped entry into the deepest part. Other forms of entry may be provided as long as a sloped entry is provided. The sloped entries for wading pools are not required to have handrails.

Spas

Spas must provide at least one accessible means of entry, which can be a pool lift, transfer wall, or transfer system. If spas are provided in a cluster, 5 percent of the total—or at least one spa—must be accessible. If there is more than one cluster, one spa or 5 percent per cluster must be accessible.

Footrests are not required on pool lifts provided at spas. However, footrests or retractable leg supports are encouraged, especially on lifts used in larger spas, where the water depth is 34 inches or more and there is sufficient space.

TYPES OF ACCESSIBLE MEANS OF ENTRY INTO THE WATER

Pool Lifts

Pool lifts must be located where the water level is not deeper than 48 inches. This provides the opportunity for someone to provide assistance from a standing position in the water if desired. If multiple pool lift locations are provided, only one must be

where the water is less than 48 inches. If the entire pool is deeper than 48 inches, an exception allows operators to use a pool lift in any location as an accessible means of entry.

Seats

There are a variety of seats available on pool lifts and these guidelines do not specify the type of material or the type of seat required. However, lift seats must be a minimum of 16 inches wide. In the raised (load) position, the centerline of the seat must be located over the deck, a minimum of 16 inches from the edge of the pool. The deck surface between the centerline of the seat and the pool edge cannot have a slope greater than 1:48.

Although not required, seats with backs will enable a larger number of persons with disabilities to use the lift independently. Pool lift seats made of materials that resist corrosion, that provide a firm base, and that are padded are more usable. Headrests, seat belts, and additional leg support may also enhance accessibility and accommodate a wider variety of people with disabilities.

Clear Deck Space

Clear deck space must be provided to enable a person to get close enough to the pool lift seat to easily transfer from a wheelchair or mobility device. This clear deck space will ensure an unobstructed area for transfers between a mobility device and the seat. The clear deck space must be a minimum of 36 inches wide and extend forward a minimum of 48 inches from a line located 12 inches behind the

12 in. from back edge of seat

16 in.-19 in. seat height above pool deck

36 in. minimum

48 in. minimum

Pool lift.

rear edge of the seat. This space must be located on the side of the seat opposite the water. The slope of the clear deck space must not be greater than 1:48 (2 percent). This virtually flat area will make the transfer easier and safer, while still allowing water to drain away from the deck.

Seat Height

The lift must be designed so that the seat will make a stop between a minimum of 16 inches and maximum of 19 inches (measured from the deck to the top of the seat surface, when the seat is in the raised position). Lifts can provide additional stops at various heights to accommodate users of all ages and abilities.

Footrests and Armrests

Footrests and armrests provide stability for the person using the pool lift. Footrests must be provided on pool lifts, and must move together with the seat. Padding on footrests—large enough to support the whole foot—reduces the chance of injury.

Armrests are not required; however if provided, the armrest opposite the water must be removable or be able to fold clear of the seat when the seat is in the raised (load) position. This clearance is needed for people transferring between the lift and a mobility device.

Operation

Lifts must be designed and placed so that people can use them without assistance, although assistance can be provided if needed. A person must be able

Pool lift submerged depth.

to call the lift when it is in either the deck or water position. It is especially important for someone who is swimming alone to be able to call the lift so she or he won't be stranded in the water for an extended period of time.

The controls and operating mechanisms must be unobstructed when a lift is in use. A person must be able to use the lift with one hand, and the operating controls must not require tight grasping, pinching, or twisting of the wrist. Controls may not require more than five pounds of pressure to operate.

Submerged Depth

Lifts must be designed so that the seat will submerge to a minimum of 18 inches below the stationary water level. This will ensure buoyancy for the person on the lift and make it easier to enter or exit.

Lifting Capacity

Lifts must have the capability of supporting a minimum weight of 300 pounds and be capable of sustaining a static load that is at least 1.5 times the rated load. Where possible, lifts that can support a greater weight capacity are encouraged.

SLOPED ENTRIES

Sloped entries must comply with ADAAG accessible route provisions (36 inch minimum width, maximum 1:12 or 8.33 percent slope), except that the surface does not need to be slip resistant. The slope may be designed as zero grade beach or ramp access. With either design, the maximum slope permitted is 1:12 (8.33 percent).

In most cases, it is not appropriate to submerge personal wheelchairs and mobility devices in water. Some have batteries, motors, and electrical systems that can be damaged or contaminate the pool. Facilities that use sloped entries are encouraged to provide an aquatic wheelchair designed for access into the water. Persons transfer to the aquatic wheelchair and access the water using it, leaving their personal mobility device on the deck. Operators and facility managers may need to consider storage options for personal mobility devices if deck space is limited.

Submerged Depth

Sloped entries must extend to a depth between 24 inches minimum and 30 inches maximum below the stationary water level. This depth is necessary for individuals using the sloped entry to become buoyant. Where the sloped entry has a running slope greater than 1:20 (5 percent), a landing at both the

Sloped entry ramp.

top and bottom of the ramp is required. At least one landing must be located between 24 and 30 inches below the stationary water level. Landings must be a minimum of 36 inches in width and 60 inches in length. The sloped entry may be a maximum of 30 feet at 1:12 (8.33%) slope before an intermediate landing is required. Adding a solid wall on the side closest to the water can enhance safety.

Handrails

Sloped entries must have handrails on both sides regardless of the slope. Handrail extensions are required at the top landing but not at the bottom. The clear width between handrails must be between 33 and 38 inches. The handrail height must be between 34 and 48 inches to the top of the gripping surface. This provision does not require the handrails to be below the stationary water level, which could be considered an underwater obstruction. No minimum width is required between handrails provided on sloped entries that serve wave action pools, leisure rivers, sand bottom pools, and other pools where people can enter only in one place. Handrails are required to comply with ADAAG provisions (diameter, non-rotating, and height).

TRANSFER WALLS

A transfer wall is a wall along an accessible route that allows a person to leave a mobility device and transfer onto the wall and then into a pool or spa.

Grab Bars

Transfer walls must have at least one grab bar. Grab bars must be perpendicular to the pool wall and extend the full width of the wall so a person can use them for support into the water. The top of the gripping surface must be 4 to 6 inches above the wall to provide leverage to the person using the bars. If only one bar is provided, the clearance must be a minimum of 24 inches on each side of the bar. If two bars are provided, the clearance must be a minimum of 24 inches between the bars. The diameter of the grab bars must comply with ADAAG (diameter between 1.25 and 1.5 inches, not abrasive, and non-rotating).

Clear Deck Space

Clear deck space of 60 by 60 inches minimum, with a slope of not more than 1:48, must be provided at the base of a transfer wall. This will allow persons using a wheelchair to turn around and access the

Transfer wall with one grab bar.

Transfer wall with two grab bars.

wall, depending on the side they can best use to transfer. If there is one grab bar on a transfer wall, the clear deck space must be centered on the one grab bar. That allows enough space for a transfer on either side of the bar. If two bars are provided, the clear deck space must be centered on the 24-inch clearance between the two bars.

Height

The transfer wall height must be 16 inches minimum to 19 inches maximum, measured from the deck.

Width and Length

Transfer walls must be a minimum of 12 inches wide to a maximum of 16 inches wide. This provides enough space for a person to sit comfortably on the surface of the wall and pivot to access the water. The wall must be a minimum of 60 inches long and must be centered on the clear deck space. Additional length will provide increased space and options for transferring.

Surface

Since people using transfer walls are in bathing suits, their skin may be in contact with the wall. To prevent injuries, the wall surface must have rounded edges and not be sharp.

TRANSFER SYSTEMS

A transfer system consists of a transfer platform and a series of transfer steps that descend into the water. Users need to transfer from their wheelchair or mobility device to the transfer platform and continue transferring into the water, step by step, bumping their way in or out of the pool.

Transfer Platform

Each transfer system must have a platform on the deck surface so users can maneuver on and off the system from their mobility device or wheelchair. Platforms must be a minimum of 19 inches deep by 24 inches wide. That provides enough room for a person transferring to maintain balance and provides enough space to maneuver on top of it.

Platform Height

Transfer platforms must be between 16 and 19 inches high, measured from the deck.

Clear Deck Space

The base of the transfer platform must have a clear deck space adjacent to it that is 60 by 60 inches minimum, with a slope not steeper than 1:48 so a person using a wheelchair can turn around and maneuver into transfer position. The space must be centered along the 24-inch minimum unobstructed side of the transfer platform. A level, unobstructed space will help a person transferring from a mobility device.

Transfer Steps

The maximum height of transfer steps is 8 inches, although shorter heights are recommended. Each transfer step must have a tread depth of 14 inches minimum to 17 inches maximum and a minimum tread width of 24 inches. The steps must extend into the water a minimum of 18 inches below the stationary water level.

Surface

The surface of the transfer platform and steps must not be sharp and must have rounded edges to prevent injuries.

Transfer system platform and steps.

Clear deck space located at a transfer system.

Grab Bars

A grab bar must be provided on at least one side of each step and on the transfer platform, or as a continuous grab bar serving each step and the platform. The bar must not obstruct transfer onto the platform. If a grab bar is provided on each step, the top of the gripping surface must be 4 inches minimum to 6 inches maximum above each step. If a continuous bar is provided, the top of the gripping surface must be 4 inches minimum to 6 inches maximum above each step nosing. Grab bars on transfer systems must comply with ADAAG (diameter between 1.25 and 1.5 inches, not abrasive, and non-rotating).

Continuous grab bar at transfer system.

ACCESSIBLE POOL STAIRS

Accessible pool stairs are designed to provide assistance with balance and support from a standing position when moving from the pool deck into the water and out. ADAAG provisions for stairs include the requirement that all steps have uniform riser heights and uniform tread widths of not less than 11 inches, measured from riser to riser. Additionally, open risers are not permitted. Other stairs or steps provided in the pool are not required to meet these guidelines.

Pool stairs.

Handrails

Pool stairs must have handrails with a minimum width between the rails of 20 inches and a maximum of 24 inches. The 20- to 24-inch width for the accessible pool stairs is intended to provide support for individuals with disabilities who are ambulatory. Handrail extensions are required on the top landing of the stairs but are not required at the bottom landing. Handrails on pool stairs must comply with ADAAG provisions. The top of the handrail gripping surface must be a minimum of 34 inches and a maximum of 38 inches above the stair nosing. If handrails are mounted on walls, the clear space between the handrail and wall must be 1.5 inches.

WATER PLAY COMPONENTS

If water play components are provided, they must comply with the Access Board's Play Area Guidelines and accessible route provisions.

If the surface of the accessible route, clear floor or ground spaces, and turning spaces that connect play components are submerged, the accessible route does not have to comply with the requirements for cross slope, running slope, and surface conditions.

Transfer systems may be used instead of ramps to connect elevated water play components.

OTHER ACCESSIBLE ELEMENTS

If swimming pools are part of a multiuse facility, designers and operators must also comply with ADAAG and all applicable requirements for recreation facilities. These include, but are not limited to:

- Dressing, fitting, and locker rooms
- Exercise equipment and machines
- Areas of sports activities (court sports, sports fields, etc.)
- Play areas
- Saunas and steam rooms

MORE INFORMATION

You can obtain copies of the recreation facility guidelines, which include swimming pools, wading pools, and spas, and further technical assistance from the U.S. Access Board at www.access-board. gov, 1-800-872-2253, or 1-800-993-2822 (TTY).

Trade and Professional Associations Involved in the Health/Fitness Facility Industry

Aerobics and Fitness Association of America
15250 Ventura Boulevard, Suite 200
Sherman Oaks, CA 91403
877-968-7263
www.afaa.com

American Association of Cardiovascular
and Pulmonary Rehabilitation
401 North Michigan Avenue, Suite 2200
Chicago, IL 60611
312-321-5146
www.aacvpr.org

American Alliance for Health, Physical
Education, Recreation and Dance
1900 Association Drive
Reston, VA 20191
800-213-7193
www.aahperd.org

American College of Sports Medicine
401 West Michigan Street
P.O. Box 1440
Indianapolis, IN 46206-1440
317-637-9200
www.acsm.org

American Council on Exercise
4851 Paramount Drive
San Diego, CA 92123
800-825-3636
www.acefitness.org

American Heart Association
7272 Greenville Avenue
Dallas, TX 75231
800-242-8721
www.americanheart.org

American Massage Therapy Association
500 Davis Street, Suite 900
Evanston, IL 60201-4444
877-905-2700
www.amta-wa.org

IDEA Health and Fitness Association
10455 Pacific Center Court
San Diego, CA 92121-4339
800-999-4332
www.ideafit.com

International Health, Racquet and Sportclub Association
263 Summer Street
Boston, MA 02210
800-228-4772
www.ihrsa.org

National Athletic Trainers Association
2952 Stemmons Freeway
Dallas, TX 75247
214-637-6282
www.nata.org

National Institute for Occupational Safety and Health
Hubert Humphrey Building
200 Independence Avenue, SW
Washington, DC 20201
800-356-4674
www.cdc.gov/niosh

National Strength and Conditioning Association
1885 Bob Johnson Drive
Colorado Springs, CO 80906
800-815-6826
www.nsca-lift.org

National Swimming Pool Association
4775 Granby Circle
Colorado Springs, CO 80919-3131
www.nspf.com

National Wellness Institute
1300 College Court
P.O. Box 827
Stevens Point, WI 54481
800-243-8694
www.nationalwellness.org

President's Council on Physical Fitness and Sports
200 Independence Avenue, SW
Room 738–H
Washington, DC 20201-0004
202-690-9000
www.fitness.gov

Sporting Goods Manufacturing Association
1150 17th Street, NW #850
Washington, DC 20036
202-775-1762
www.sgma.com

U.S. Squash Racquets Association
P.O. Box 1216
Bala Cynwyd, PA 19004
610-667-4006
www.us-squash.org

Wellness Councils of America
9802 Nicholas Street
Suite 315
Omaha, NE 68114
402-827-3590
www.welcoa.org

About the American College of Sports Medicine

"Advancing health through science, education and medicine."

This simple statement describes a complex organization working to improve quality of life in more than 80 countries. The American College of Sports Medicine is more than 20,000 professionals practicing clinical medicine, research, education, and an array of health and fitness disciplines.

The world's largest organization of its kind, ACSM tackles issues as diverse as obesity and motorsport injuries. The College is at the nexus of science and public policy, working to develop new knowledge and apply it toward a healthier, more fit society. From astronauts to student-athletes, physiologists to personal trainers, people turn to ACSM for definitive information on health, fitness, sports medicine, and exercise science. Founded in 1954, ACSM is internationally regarded as defining the gold standard for science, education, and certification.

ACSM reaches professionals and the public through a variety of means:

- Periodicals such as *Medicine & Science in Sports & Exercise®*, *Sports Medicine Bulletin*, *Exercise and Sport Sciences® Reviews*, *ACSM's Health & Fitness Journal®*, and the online consumer newsletter *ACSM Fit Society®* Page.
- The ACSM Web site, www.acsm.org, serves as a portal to health and fitness information, science-based guidance, professional development, and other resources.
- Meetings present the latest scientific research and practical and clinical applications as well as fitness techniques and public health issues.
- Through media outreach, ACSM experts provide accurate, evidence-based insight into sports medicine, exercise science, and health and fitness.
- Books, pamphlets, and other publications present consumer advice, standards and guidelines for practitioners, and other definitive information.

ACSM MEMBERSHIP

The American College of Sports Medicine is a lifelong resource, serving student members and working professionals in more than 50 occupations. ACSM membership brings a host of benefits, such as publications, conferences, and regional chapter services. Members enjoy special discounts and opportunities.

Membership categories include the following:

- Professional member (degreed or working in a relevant field)
- Professional-in-training member (in residency or postdoctoral fellowship)

- Associate member (interested in sports medicine or exercise science; not eligible for other membership categories)
- Graduate student member
- Undergraduate student member
- ACSM'S Alliance of Health and Fitness Professionals (professionals or students in the health and fitness and medical fitness industries)

And, in recognition of their distinguished achievement and service to the profession, members can pursue the status of Fellow in the American College of Sports Medicine

As professionals in training, students are an important focus of ACSM. The board of trustees includes student representation, and each Regional Chapter selects a representative to the Student Affairs Committee. *ACSM's Online Graduate and Undergraduate Programs Link* connects students with academic programs at colleges and universities. Student members enjoy discounted dues, publications, and meetings.

ACSM CERTIFICATION: THE GOLD STANDARD

ACSM's emphasis on rigorous science and professionalism has earned it a reputation as the gold standard for certification of health and fitness professionals. To consumers, institutions, and organizations that insist on demonstrated knowledge, skills, and abilities, ACSM certification signifies the highest level of preparation and practice.

For more on ACSM certification programs, see the section *ACSM Certification Programs*, in the next column.

ACSM INTEREST GROUPS

Interest Groups provide a forum for focused discussion, activity, and debate among members with similar interests. Many find the networking opportunities especially valuable. Through participation in ACSM Interest Groups, members take part in the academic and professional life of the College and help advance its mission.

ACSM REGIONAL CHAPTERS

Twelve Regional Chapters allow greater participation among members and encourage networking and professional growth for longtime members and students alike. Regional C1hapters produce publications and hold annual scientific meetings.

CONTACTING ACSM

www.acsm.org
P.O. Box 1440
Indianapolis, IN 46206-1440
317-637-9200 (phone)
317-634-7817 (fax)

AMERICAN COLLEGE OF SPORTS MEDICINE CERTIFICATIONS FOR HEALTH AND FITNESS PROFESSIONALS

For 30 years, professionals who wish to demonstrate the highest level of expertise in exercise testing and prescription have sought ACSM certification. This gold standard distinguishes those who work in many settings:

- Hospital clinical and rehabilitation programs
- Corporate wellness centers
- Park and recreation departments
- Health and fitness facilities
- Senior residences and care programs

ACSM CERTIFICATION PROGRAMS

The American College of Sports Medicine offers the following credentials:

- ACSM certified Personal Trainer℠ (cPT)
- ACSM Health/Fitness Instructor® (HFI)
- ACSM Exercise Specialist® (ES)
- ACSM Registered Clinical Exercise Physiologist® (RCEP)

The ACSM certified Personal Trainer℠ is a fitness professional involved in developing and implementing an individualized approach to exercise leadership in healthy populations and in those with medical clearance to exercise. Using a variety of teaching techniques, the Personal Trainer is proficient in leading and demonstrating safe and effective methods of exercise by applying the principles of exercise science. The ACSM certified Personal Trainer℠ is familiar with forms of exercise used to improve, maintain, and optimize health-related components of physical fitness and performance. Personal Trainers are proficient in writing appropriate exercise recommendations, leading and demonstrating safe and effective methods of exercise, and motivating people to begin and to continue with their healthy behaviors.

The ACSM Health/Fitness Instructor® (HFI) is a professional qualified to assess, design, and implement individual and group exercise and fitness programs for low-risk individuals and individuals with controlled disease. The HFI is skilled in evaluating health behaviors and risk factors, conducting fitness assessments, writing appropriate exercise prescriptions, and motivating individuals to modify negative health habits and maintain positive lifestyle behaviors for health promotion.

The ACSM Exercise Specialist® (ES) is a healthcare professional certified by ACSM to deliver a variety of services in exercise assessment, training, rehabilitation, risk-factor identification, and lifestyle management to people with or at risk for cardiovascular, pulmonary, and metabolic diseases. These services typically are delivered in cardiovascular and pulmonary rehabilitation programs, physicians' offices, and medical fitness centers. The ACSM Exercise Specialist also is qualified to provide exercise-related consulting for research, public health, and other clinical and nonclinical services and programs.

The ACSM Registered Clinical Exercise Physiologist® (RCEP) is an allied health professional who works with persons with chronic diseases and conditions in which exercise has been shown to be beneficial. The RCEP performs health, physical activity, and fitness assessments and prescribes exercise and physical activity primarily in hospitals or other health-provider settings.

Certification at a given level requires the candidate to have a knowledge and skills base commensurate with that specific level of certification. In addition, the HFI level of certification incorporates the knowledge, skills, and abilities (KSAs) associated with the ACSM certified Personal Trainer℠ certification. ES certification incorporates the KSAs associated with HFI certification. Each level of certification has minimum requirements for experience, level of education, and other certifications.

30 YEARS OF CERTIFICATION

The ACSM certification program began in 1975 along with publication of the first edition of *ACSM's Guidelines for Exercise Testing and Prescription*. That era was marked by rapid development of exercise programs for patients with stable coronary artery disease (CAD). ACSM sought a means to disseminate accurate information on this health-care initiative through expression of consensus from its members in basic science, clinical practice, and education. These early clinical certifications helped establish safe and scientifically based exercise services for cardiac rehabilitation.

Over the past 30 years, exercise has gained widespread recognition as an important component in programs of rehabilitative care or health maintenance for an expanding list of chronic diseases and disabling conditions. The growth of public interest in the role of exercise in health promotion has been equally impressive. In addition, federal policy makers have revisited questions of medical efficacy and financing for exercise services in rehabilitative care of selected patients. Over the past several years, recommendations from the U.S. Public Health Service and the U.S. Surgeon General have acknowledged the central role that regular physical activity can play in preventing disease and promoting health.

ACSM's development of the health and fitness certifications in the 1980s increased the availability of qualified professionals providing scientifically sound advice and supervision regarding physical activities in apparently healthy adults. Since 1975, ACSM has certified more than 30,000 professionals. Many colleges and universities have adopted ACSM guidelines in establishing standardized curricula that are focused on the knowledge, skills, and abilities (KSAs) required for certification as Health/Fitness Instructor®, ACSM Exercise Specialist® or ACSM Registered Clinical Exercise Physiologist®. The ACSM University Connection Endorsement program is designed to recognize institutions with educational programs that meet all of the KSAs specified by the ACSM Committee on Certification and Registry Boards (CCRB).

ACSM's Certified News brings best practices and other information to certified professionals. ACSM also oversees continuing education requirements for maintenance of certification. Continuing education credits can be accrued through ACSM-sponsored educational programs such as workshops (ACSM Health/Fitness Instructor® and ACSM Exercise Specialist®), Regional Chapter meetings and annual meetings, and other educational programs approved by the ACSM Professional Education Committee. These enhancements support the continued professional growth of those who have made a commitment to service in the health and fitness field.

HOW TO OBTAIN INFORMATION AND APPLICATION MATERIALS

ACSM certification programs are subject to continual review and revision. Content development is entrusted to a diverse committee of professional volunteers with expertise in exercise science, medicine, and program management. The committee's expertise also includes design and procedures for competency assessment. The ACSM National Center oversees administration of certification. Inquiries concerning certifications, application requirements, fees, and examination test sites and dates may be made to:

ACSM Certification Resource Center
1-800-486-5643
Web site: www.lww.com/acsmcrc
E-mail: certification@acsm.org

AHA/ACSM Joint Position Statement

Recommendations for Cardiovascular Screening, Staffing, and Emergency Policies at Health/Fitness Facilities

SUMMARY

The promotion of physical activity is at the top of our national public health agenda. Although regular exercise reduces subsequent cardiovascular morbidity and mortality, the incidence of a cardiovascular event during exercise in patients with cardiac disease is estimated to be 10 times that of otherwise healthy persons. Adequate screening and evaluation are important to identify and counsel persons with underlying cardiovascular disease before they begin exercising at moderate to vigorous levels. This statement provides recommendations for *cardiovascular screening* of all persons (children, adolescents, and adults) before enrollment or participation in activities at health/fitness facilities. Staff qualifications and emergency policies related to cardiovascular safety are also discussed.

INTRODUCTION

The message from the nation's scientists is clear, unequivocal, and unified: physical inactivity is a risk factor for cardiovascular disease (7,18), and its prevalence is an important public health issue. New scientific knowledge based on epidemiological observational studies, cohort studies, controlled trials, and basic research has led to an unprecedented focus on physical activity and exercise. The promotion of physical activity is at the top of our national public health agenda, as seen in the publication of the 1996 report of the U.S. Surgeon General on physical activity and health (20).

The attention now being given to physical activity supports the goals of Healthy People 2000 (10) and should lead to increased levels of regular physical activity throughout the U.S. population, including the nearly one fourth of adult Americans who have some form of cardiovascular disease (3). Although regular exercise reduces subsequent cardiovascular morbidity and mortality (7,17,18), the incidence of a cardiovascular event during exercise in patients with cardiac disease is estimated to be 10 times that of otherwise healthy persons (8). Adequate screening and evaluation are important to identify and counsel persons with underlying cardiovascular disease before they begin exercising at moderate to vigorous levels.

Moderate (or higher) levels of physical activity and exercise are achieved in a number of settings, including more than 15,000 health/fitness facilities across the country. A recent survey of 110 health/fitness facilities in Massachusetts found that efforts to screen new members at enrollment were limited and inconsistent (14). Nearly 40% of responding facilities stated that they do not routinely use a screening interview or questionnaire to evaluate new members for symptoms or history of cardiovascular disease, and 10% stated that they conducted no initial cardiovascular health history screening at all.

This statement provides recommendations for *cardiovascular screening* of all persons (children, adolescents, and adults) before enrollment or participation in activities at health/fitness facilities. Staff qualifications and emergency policies related to cardiovascular safety are also discussed. Health/fitness facilities are defined here as organizations that offer health and fitness programs as their primary or secondary service or that promote high-intensity recreational physical activity (e.g., basketball, tennis, racquetball, and swim clubs). Ideally such facilities have a professional staff, but those that provide space and equipment only (e.g., unsupervised hotel exercise rooms) are also included. A health/fitness facility user is defined as a dues-paying member or a guest paying a regular daily fee to use the facility specifically to exercise. These recommendations are intended to assist health/fitness facility staff, healthcare providers, and consumers in the promotion and performance of safe and effective physical activity/exercise.

The writing group based these recommendations on a review of the literature and the consensus of the group. Earlier statements from the American Heart Association (AHA) and the American College of Sports Medicine (ACSM) are highlighted and supplemented. These recommendations were peer reviewed by selected authorities in the field representing the AHA, the ACSM, the American College of Cardiology, the International Health Racquet and Sports Clubs Association (IHRSA), and the Young Men's Christian Association. The recommendations are not mandatory or all-encompassing, nor do they limit provision of individualized care by practitioners exercising independent judgment. With this statement the AHA and the ACSM assume no responsibility toward any individual for whom this statement may be applied in the provision of individualized care. Specific details about exercise testing and training of persons with and without

cardiovascular disease and those with other health problems are provided elsewhere (2,6,8,21). The ACSM has published comprehensive guidelines for operating health/fitness facilities (19). Although issues in competitive sports are beyond the scope of this statement, the 26th Bethesda Conference (28) on sudden cardiac death in competitive athletes and the AHA (12) provide specific recommendations for the screening and evaluation of athletes for congenital heart disease, systemic hypertension, and other cardiovascular diseases before participation in competitive sports.

CARDIOVASCULAR SCREENING

Rationale

Regular exercise results in increased exercise capacity and physical fitness, which can lead to many health benefits. Persons who are physically active appear to have lower rates of all-cause mortality, probably because of a decrease in occurrence of chronic illnesses, including coronary heart disease. This benefit may be the result of an improvement in cardiovascular risk factors in addition to enhanced fibrinolysis, improved endothelial function, decreased sympathetic tone, and other as yet undetermined factors (7). Regular endurance exercise leads to favorable alterations in the cardiovascular, musculoskeletal, and neurohumoral systems. The result is a training effect, which allows an individual to do increasing amounts of work while lowering the heart rate and blood pressure response to submaximal exercise. Such an effect is particularly desirable in patients with coronary artery disease because it allows increased activity with less ischemia (7).

The Centers for Disease Control and Prevention (18), the ACSM (18), and the AHA (6) recommend that every American participate in at least moderate-intensity physical activity for ≥30 min on most, if not all, days of the week. Unfortunately, many Americans are sedentary or perform too little physical activity; only 22% of adult Americans engage in regular exercise ≥5 times a week (20). The prevalence of physical inactivity is higher among culturally diverse segments of the U.S. population, low-income groups, the elderly, and women (20). It is important for healthcare providers to educate the public about the benefits of physical activity and to encourage more leisure-time exercise, particularly for those who are underactive. Consumers should seek information about safe and effective ways to increase physical activity and initiate and maintain a regular program of exercise.

Efforts to promote physical activity will result in an increasing number of persons with and without heart disease joining the more than 20 million persons who already exercise at health/fitness facilities (16). Current market research indicates that 50% of health/fitness facility members are older than 35 yr, and the fastest-growing segments of users are those older than 55 yr and those aged 35-54 yr (16). With increased physical activity, more people with symptoms of or known cardiovascular disease will face the cardiovascular stress of physical activity and possible risk of a cardiac event. More than one fourth of all Americans have some form of cardiovascular disease (3). The prevalence of coronary heart disease for American adults aged 20 yr and older is 7.2% in the general population, 7.5% for non-Hispanic whites, 6.9% for non-Hispanic blacks, and 5.6% for Mexican Americans (3). The prevalence of myocardial infarction in older Americans aged 65-69 yr is 18.0% for men and 9.7% for women (3).

Moderately strenuous physical exertion may trigger ischemic cardiac events, particularly among persons not accustomed to regular physical activity and exercise. Siscovick et al. (23) examined the incidence of primary cardiac arrest in men aged 25-75 yr after excluding those with a history of clinically recognized heart disease. Although the risk was significantly increased during high-intensity exercise, the likelihood for primary cardiac arrest during such activity in a clinically healthy population was estimated at 0.55 events/10,000 men per year. Maron et al. (13) studied causes of sudden death in competitive athletes. In persons younger than 35 yr, 48% of deaths were due to hypertrophic cardiomyopathy. Coronary artery anomalies, idiopathic left ventricular hypertrophy, and coronary heart disease each accounted for 10-20% of deaths. In those over 35, coronary artery disease accounted for approximately 80% of all deaths. Overall, the absolute incidence of death during exercise in the general population is low (25,26,29). *Each year approximately 0.75 and 0.13/100,000 young male and female athletes (29) and 6/100,000 middle-aged men die during exertion (25).* No estimates are available for middle-aged women or the elderly.

Cardiovascular events other than death during exercise have also been studied. Data from the Framingham heart study indicate that the baseline risk of myocardial infarction in a 50-yr-old man who is a nonsmoker and does not have diabetes is approximately 1% per year, or approximately 1 chance per million per hour (4). Heavy exertion [≥6 METs (metabolic equivalents)] within 1 h of symptomatic onset of acute myocardial infarction has been reported in 4.4-7.1% of patients (15,31). The adjusted relative risk is significantly greater in persons who do not participate in regular physical activity, with an approximate threefold increase in risk during the morning hours. The relation of physical activity to acute myocardial infarction in the thrombolytic era was examined among 3339 patients in the TIMI II trial (27), in which moderate or marked physical activity preceded myocardial infarction in 18.7% of patients.

Van Camp et al. (30) reported the incidence of major cardiovascular complications in 167 randomly selected cardiac rehabilitation programs that provided supervised exercise training to 51,000 patients with known cardiovascular disease. The incidence of myocardial infarction was 1 per 294,000 person-hours; the incidence of death was 1 per 784,000 person-hours.

Screening Prospective Members/Users

All facilities offering exercise equipment or services should conduct cardiovascular screening of all new members and/or prospective users. The primary purpose of preparticipation screening is to identify both those not known to be at risk and those known to be at risk for a cardiovascular event during exercise. Recent evidence suggests that screening by health/fitness facilities is done only sporadically (14). In Canada, evidence from the Canadian Home Fitness test and its screening instrument, the Physical Activity Readiness Questionnaire (PAR-Q), suggests that even simple screening questionnaires can effectively identify many persons at high risk and increase the safety of nonsupervised exercise (22). Current knowledge of the relation between identifiable risk factors, the incidence of cardiovascular disease, and the triggering factors for acute myocardial infarction suggests that screening is both reasonable and prudent.

The cost-effectiveness of preparticipation screening is an important consideration. Exercise testing is comparatively expensive. The incidence of false-positive findings when testing asymptomatic persons (9) and the need to follow up abnormal results can lead to subsequent and more costly procedures. A thorough and mandatory screening process that might prove optimally sensitive in detecting occult cardiovascular disease might be so prohibitive to participation that fewer persons would engage in a fitness program. Such a result would be counterproductive to the goal of maximizing physical activity. Because most of the health benefits of exercise accrue at moderate levels of intensity (18), in which the risks are probably low, recommendations that would inhibit large numbers of persons from participating in exercise programs are not justified. Preparticipation screening should identify persons at high risk and should be simple and easy to perform. Public health efforts should focus on increasing the use of preparticipation screening.

Two practical tools for preparticipation screening are likely to have an effect on identifying high-risk individuals without inhibiting their participation in exercise programs. The PAR-Q (24) (Table 1) is a self-administered questionnaire that focuses primarily on symptoms that might suggest angina pectoris. Participants are directed to contact their personal physician if they answer "yes" to ≥1 questions. The PAR-Q also identifies musculoskeletal problems that should be evaluated before participation because these might involve modification of the exercise program. The questionnaire is designed to be completed when the participant registers at a health/fitness facility. In unsupervised fitness facilities (e.g., hotel fitness centers), the PAR-Q can be self-administered by means of signs prominently displayed at the main entry into the facility. Although less satisfactory than documenting the results of screening, use of signs and similar visual methods are a minimal recommendation for encouraging prospective users to assess their health risks while exercising at any facility.

Another simple, self-administered device that aims to identify high-risk individuals without negatively impacting participation is a questionnaire patterned after one developed by the Wisconsin Affiliate of the American Heart Association (11) (Table 2). The one-page form is slightly more complex than the PAR-Q and uses history, symptoms, and risk factors (including age) to direct prospective members to either participate in an exercise program or contact their physician (or appropriate healthcare provider) before participation. Persons at higher risk are directed to seek facilities providing appropriate levels of staff supervision. The questionnaire can be administered within a few minutes on the same form participants use to join or register at the facility. It identifies potentially high-risk participants, documents the results of screening, educates the consumer, and encourages and fosters appropriate use of the healthcare system. In addition, it can guide staff qualifications and requirements. This instrument is also simple enough to be adapted for use as self-screening signs posted in nonstaffed facilities.

Health appraisal questionnaires should preferably be interpreted by qualified staff (see next section for criteria) who can limit the number of unnecessary referrals for preparticipation medical evaluation, avoiding undue expense and barriers to participation.

In view of the potential legal risk assumed by operators of health/fitness facilities, it is recommended that all facilities providing staff supervision document the results of screening. Screening, particularly for participants for whom a medical evaluation is recommended, requires time, personnel, and financial resources. Individual facilities can determine the most cost-effective way to conduct and document preparticipation screening.

Every effort should be made to educate all prospective new members about the importance of obtaining a health appraisal and—*if indicated*—medical evaluation/recommendation before beginning exercise testing/training. The potential risks

TABLE 1   Revised Physical Activity Readiness Questionnaire (PAR-Q)

Yes	No	
___	___	1. Has a doctor ever said that you have a heart condition and recommended only medically supervised activity?
___	___	2. Do you have chest pain brought on by physical activity?
___	___	3. Have you developed chest pain in the past month?
___	___	4. Have you on one or more occasions lost consciousness or fallen over as a result of dizziness?
___	___	5. Do you have a bone or joint problem that could be aggravated by the proposed physical activity?
___	___	6. Has a doctor ever recommended medication for your blood pressure or a heart condition?
___	___	7. Are you aware, through your own experience or a doctor's advice, of any other physical reason that would prohibit you from exercising without medical supervision?

If you answer "yes" to any of these questions, call your personal physician or healthcare provider before increasing your physical activity.

Adapted from Shephard et al. (22) and Thomas et al. (24).

TABLE 2   AHA/ACSM Health/Fitness Facility Preparticipation Screening Questionnaire

Assess your health needs by marking all *true* statements.

History

You have had:

_____ heart attack

_____ heart surgery

_____ cardiac catheterization

_____ pacemaker/implantable cardiac defibrillator/rhythm disturbance

_____ heart valve disease

_____ heart failure

_____ heart transplantation

_____ congenital heart disease

*If you marked any of the statements in this section, consult your healthcare provider before engaging in exercise. You may need to use a facility with a **medically qualified staff**.*

Symptoms

You have had:

_____ You experience chest discomfort with exertion.

_____ You experience unreasonable breathlessness.

_____ You experience dizziness, fainting, blackouts.

_____ You take heart medications.

Other health issues

_____ You have musculoskeletal problems.

_____ You have concerns about the safety of exercise.

_____ You take prescription medication(s).

_____ You are pregnant.

Cardiovascular risk factors

_____ You are a man older than 45 years.

_____ You are a woman older than 55 years or you have had a hysterectomy or you are postmenopausal.

_____ You smoke.

_____ Your blood pressure is greater than 140/90.

_____ You don't know your blood pressure.

_____ You take blood pressure medication.

_____ Your blood cholesterol level is >240 mg/dL.

*If you marked two or more of the statements in this section, you should consult your healthcare provider before engaging in exercise. You might benefit by using a facility with a **professionally qualified exercise staff** to guide your exercise program.*

_____ You don't know your cholesterol level.

_____ You have a close blood relative who had a heart attack before age 55 (father or brother) or age 65 (mother or sister).

_____ You are diabetic or take medicine to control your blood sugar.

_____ You are physically inactive (i.e., you get less than 30 minutes of physical activity on at least 3 days per week).

_____ You are more than 20 pounds overweight.

_____ None of the above is true.

You should be able to exercise safely without consulting your healthcare provider in almost any facility that meets your exercise program needs.

AHA/ACSM indicates American Heart Association/American College of Sports Medicine.

inherent in not obtaining an appraisal should also be emphasized. Without an appraisal, it is impossible to determine whether a person may be at significant risk of severe bodily harm or death by participating in an exercise program. The same is true of persons who undergo a health appraisal, are identified as having symptoms of or known cardiovascular disease, and refuse or neglect to obtain the recom-

mended medical evaluation yet seek admission to a health/fitness facility program. *Due to safety concerns, persons with known cardiovascular disease who do not obtain recommended medical evaluations and those who fail to complete the health appraisal questionnaire upon request may be excluded from participation in a health/fitness facility exercise program to the extent permitted by law.*

Persons without symptoms or a known history of cardiovascular disease who do not obtain the recommended medical evaluation after completing a health appraisal should be required to sign an assumption of risk or release/waiver. Both of these forms may be legally recognized in the jurisdiction where the facility is located. When appropriate guidelines are followed, it is likely that the potential benefits of physical activity will outweigh the risks. *Persons without symptoms or a known history of cardiovascular disease who do not obtain recommended medical evaluations or sign a release/waiver upon request may be excluded from participation in a health/fitness facility exercise program to the extent permitted by law. Persons who do not obtain an evaluation but who sign a release/waiver may be permitted to participate.* However, they should be encouraged to participate in only moderate- or lower-intensity physical activities and counseled about warning symptoms and signs of an impending cardiovascular event.

The major objectives of preparticipation cardiovascular screening are to identify persons with known cardiovascular disease, symptoms of cardiovascular disease, and/or risk factors for disease development who should receive a medical evaluation/recommendation before starting an exercise program or undergoing exercise testing. Screening also identifies persons with known cardiovascular disease who should not participate in an exercise program or who should participate at least initially in a medically supervised program, as well as persons with other special needs (8,19).

Screening also serves another purpose. One of the trends in cardiac rehabilitation is to "mainstream" low-risk, clinically stable patients to community facilities rather than specialized, often costly cardiac programs. Facility directors should expect that an increasing percentage of their participants will have health histories that warrant supervision of exercise programs by professional staff.

When a medical evaluation/recommendation is advised or required, written and active communication with the individual's personal physician (or healthcare provider) is strongly recommended. The sample letter and medical release form in Table 3, A and B, can be used or modified for such purposes.

TABLE 3A Sample Physician Referral Form[a]

Dear Dr.

Your patient (*name of patient*) would like to begin a program of exercise and/or sports activity at (*name of health/fitness facility*). After reviewing his/her responses to our cardiovascular screening questionnaire, we would appreciate your medical opinion and recommendations concerning his/her participation in exercise/sports activity. *Please provide the following information and return this form to (name, address, telephone, fax of health/fitness facility contact):*

1. Are there specific concerns or conditions our staff should be aware of before this individual engages in exercise/sports activity at our facility? Yes/No. If yes, please specify:

   _____

   _____

2. If this individual has completed an exercise test, please provide the following:
   a. Date of test
   b. A copy of the final exercise test report and interpretation
   c. Your specific recommendations for exercise training, including heart rate limits during exercise:

   _____

   _____

3. Please provide the following information so that we may contact you if we have any further questions:
   ____ I AGREE to the participation of this individual in exercise/sports activity at your health/fitness facility.
   ____ I DO NOT AGREE that this individual is a candidate to exercise at your health/fitness facility because

   _____

   _____

Physician's signature _____

Address _____

Telephone _____   Fax _____

Thank you for your help.

ᵃ Must be accompanied by a medical release form.

TABLE 3B Sample Authorization for Release of Medical Information

1. I hereby authorize _____ to release the following information from the medical record of

    Patient's name _____

    Address _____

    Telephone _____

    Date of birth _____

2. Information to be released: (*If specific treatment dates are not indicated, information from the most recent visit will be released.*)

    ___ Exercise test ___ Most recent history and physical exam

    ___ Most recent clinic visit ___ Consultations

    ___ Laboratory results (specify) _____

    ___ Other (specify) _____

3. Information to be released to:

    Name of person/organization _____

    Address _____

    Telephone _____

4. Purpose of disclosure information: _____

5. I do not give permission for disclosure or redisclosure of this information other than that specified above.

6. I request that this consent become invalid 90 days from the date I sign it or _____

I understand that this consent can be revoked at any time except to the extent that disclosure made in good faith has already occurred in reliance on this consent.

7. Patient's signature _____

    Date _____

    Witness (please print) _____

    Signature _____

Characteristics of Participants

Intensity of physical activity is measured through endurance- or strength-type exercise as defined in Table 4. Health appraisal questionnaires should be used before exercise testing and/or training to initially classify participants by risk for triage and preliminary decision making (Table 5), namely, apparently healthy persons (Class A-1), persons at increased risk (Classes A-2 and A-3), and persons with known cardiovascular disease (Classes B, C, and D). Apparently healthy persons of all ages and asymptomatic persons at increased risk (Classes A-1 through A-3) may participate in *moderate-intensity* exercise without first undergoing a medical examination or a medically supervised, symptom-limited exercise test. Apparently healthy younger persons (Class A-1) may also participate in *vigorous* exercise without first undergoing a medical examination and a medically supervised exercise test. It is suggested that persons classified as Class A-2 and particularly Class A-3 undergo a medical examination and possibly a maximal exercise test before engaging in vigorous exercise. All other persons (Classes B and C) should undergo a medical examination and perform a maximal exercise test before participation in moderate or vigorous exercise unless exercise is contraindicated (i.e., Class D). Data from a medical evaluation performed within 1 yr are acceptable unless clinical status has changed. Medically supervised exercise tests should be conducted in accordance with previously published guidelines (8).

Using Screening Results for Risk Stratification

With completion of the initial health appraisal and, if indicated, medical consultation and supervised exercise test, participants can be further classified for exercise training on the basis of individual characteristics detailed below. The following classifications have been modified using existing AHA (8) and ACSM (2) guidelines and are recommended (Table 5):

• *Class A: Apparently healthy.* There is no evidence of increased cardiovascular risk for exercise. This classification includes 1) "apparently healthy" younger persons (Class A-1) and 2) irrespective of age, persons who are "apparently healthy" or at "increased risk" (Classes A-2 and A-3) and who have a normal diagnostic maximal exercise test. Submaximal exercise tests are sometimes performed at health/fitness facilities where permitted by law for nondiagnostic purposes, including physical fitness assessment, exercise prescription, and monitoring of progress (2). Such testing is also useful for educating participants about exercise and for motivating them. Nondiagnostic exercise testing should be conducted only for persons in Class A and only by appropriately qualified, well-trained personnel (see section on staffing below) who are knowledgeable about indications and contraindications for exercise testing, indications for test termination, and test interpretation. All health/fitness facilities, including those where exercise testing is performed, should have an emergency plan (see section on emergency policies and procedures below) to ensure that emergencies are handled safely, efficiently, and effectively. No restrictions other than provision of basic guidelines are required for exercise training. No special supervision is required during exercise training.

TABLE 4   Classification of Physical Activity Intensity (20)

	ENDURANCE-TYPE ACTIVITY								STRENGTH-TYPE EXERCISE
	RELATIVE INTENSITY			ABSOLUTE INTENSITY (METs) IN HEALTHY ADULTS (AGE IN YR)					RELATIVE INTENSITY[a]
Intensity	$\dot{V}O_2$max (%) heart rate reserve (%)	Maximum heart rate (%)	RPE[b]	Young (20-39)	Middle-aged (40-64)	Old (65-79)	Very old (80+)	RPE	Maximum voluntary contraction (%)
Very light	<25	<30	<9	<3.0	<2.5	<2.0	<1.25	<10	<30
Light	25-44	30-49	9-10	3.0-4.7	2.5-4.4	2.0-3.5	1.26-2.2	10-11	30-49
Moderate	45-59	50-69	11-12	4.8-7.1	4.5-5.9	3.6-4.7	2.3-2.95	12-13	50-69
Hard	60-84	70-89	13-16	7.2-10.1	6.0-8.4	4.8-6.7	3.0-4.25	14-16	70-84
Very hard	>85	>90	>16	>10.2	>8.5	>6.8	>4.25	17-19	>85
Maximum[c]	100	100	20	12.0	10.0	8.0	5.0	20	100

[a] Based on 8-12 repetitions for persons <50 yr old and 10-15 repetitions for persons aged 50 and older.
[b] Borg rating of Relative Perceived Exertion (RPE), 6-20 scale (5).
[c] Maximum values are mean values achieved during maximum exercise by healthy adults. Absolute intensity (metabolic equivalents [METs]) values are approximate mean values for men. Mean values for women are approximately 1 to 2 METs lower than those for men.

TABLE 5 Participant/Health-Fitness Facility Selection Chart

Participant characteristics	Risk class A-1	Risk class A-2	Risk class A-3	Risk class B	Risk class C	Risk class D
Age/gender	Children	Men >45 yr	Men >45 yr	Children[a]	Children[a]	Children[a]
	Adolescents	Women >55 yr	Women >55 yr	Adolescents[a]	Adolescents[a]	Adolescents[a]
	Men <45 yr			Men	Men	Men
	Women <55 yr			Women	Women	Women
Cardiovascular risk factors	None	None	≥ 2	May be present	May be present	May be present
Known CVD	None	None	None	Yes	Yes	Yes
CVD features (see text for details)	Class A apparently healthy	Class A apparently healthy	Class A apparently healthy	Class B known CVD: low risk	Class C known CVD: moderate risk	Class D known CVD: high risk
Low intensity	Facility 1-4	Facility 1-4	Facility 1-4	Facility 1-5	Facility 4-5	Not recommended
Moderate intensity	Facility 1-4	Facility 1-4	Facility 1-4	Facility 4-5	Facility 5	Not recommended
Vigorous intensity	Facility 1-4	Facility 1-4	Facility 1-4	Facility 4-5	Facility 5	Not recommended

FACILITY CHARACTERISTICS

	Level 1	Level 2	Level 3	Level 4	Level 6
Type of facility	Unsupervised exercise room	Single exercise leader	Fitness center for healthy clients	Fitness center serving clinical populations	Medically supervised clinical exercise program
Personnel	None	• Exercise leader • Recommended: medical liaison	• General manager • Health/fitness instructor • Exercise leader • Recommended: medical liaison	• General manager • Exercise specialist • Health/fitness instructor • Medical liaison	• General manager • Exercise specialist • Health/fitness instructor • Medical liaison
Emergency plan	Present	Present	Present	Present	Present
Emergency equipment	• Telephone in room • Signs	• Telephone • Signs • Recommended: blood pressure kit; stethoscope	• Telephone • Signs • Recommended: blood pressure kit; stethoscope	• Telephone • Signs • Blood pressure kit • Stethoscope	• Telephone • Signs • Blood pressure kit • Stethoscope • Oxygen • Crash cart • Defibrillator

[a] Risk stratification for patients with congenital heart disease should be guided by recommendations of the 26th Bethesda Conference (28). CVD indicates cardiovascular disease.

• *Class B: Presence of known, stable cardiovascular disease with low risk for vigorous exercise but slightly greater than for apparently healthy persons.* This classification includes clinically stable persons with 1) coronary artery disease (myocardial infarction, coronary artery bypass surgery, percutaneous transluminal coronary angioplasty, angina pectoris, abnormal exercise test, or abnormal coronary angiogram); 2) valvular heart disease; 3) congenital heart disease (risk stratification for patients with congenital heart disease should be guided by the 26th Bethesda Conference recommendations (28)); 4) cardiomyopathy (includes stable patients with heart failure with characteristics as outlined below but not recent myocarditis or hypertrophic cardiomyopathy); and 5) exercise test abnormalities that do not meet the criteria outlined in Class C below. The clinical characteristics of such persons are 1) New York Heart Association (NYHA) Class I or II (Table 6); 2) exercise capacity >6 METs; 3) no evidence of heart failure; 4) free of ischemia or angina at rest or on the exercise test ≤ 6 METs; 5) appropriate rise in systolic blood pressure during exercise; 6) absence of nonsustained or sustained ventricular tachycardia; and 7) ability to satisfactorily self-monitor intensity of activity. For these persons, activity should be individualized with exercise prescription by qualified personnel. Medical supervision is recommended during prescription sessions and nonmedical supervision by appropriately qualified staff for other exercise sessions until the participant understands how to monitor his or her own activity. Subsequent exercise training may be performed without special supervision.

• *Class C: Those at moderate to high risk for cardiac complications during exercise and/or who are unable to self-regulate activity or understand the recommended activity level.* This classification includes persons with 1) coronary artery disease with the clinical characteristics outlined below; 2) acquired valvular heart disease; 3) congenital heart disease (risk stratification for patients with congenital heart disease should be guided by the 26th Bethesda Conference recommendations (28)); 4) cardiomyopathy (includes stable patients with heart failure with characteristics as outlined below but not recent myocarditis or hypertrophic cardiomyopathy); 5) exercise test abnormalities not directly related to ischemia; 6) a previous episode of ventricular fibrillation or cardiac arrest that did not occur in the presence of an acute ischemic event or cardiac procedure; 7) complex ventricular arrhythmias that are uncontrolled at mild to moderate work intensity with medication; 8) three-vessel or left main coronary artery disease; and 9) ejection fraction < 30%. One or more of the following clinical characteristics are also present: 1) two or more previous myocardial infarctions; 2) NYHA Class III or greater; 3) exercise capacity < 6 METs; 4) ischemic horizontal or down-sloping ST depression ≥ 1 mm or angina at a workload ≤ 6 METs; 5) a fall in systolic blood pressure with exercise; 6) a medical problem that the physician believes may be potentially life-threatening; 7) a previous episode of primary cardiac arrest; and 8) ventricular tachycardia at a workload < 6 METs. Physical activity should be individualized, and exercise should be prescribed by appropriately qualified medical personnel. Medical supervision, monitoring for adverse signs and symptoms, electrocardiographic monitoring of heart rate and rhythm, and blood pressure monitoring are recommended during exercise sessions until safety is established. Subsequent exercise training should be supervised by appropriately qualified personnel.

• *Class D: Unstable conditions with activity restriction.* This classification includes those with 1) unstable ischemia; 2) heart failure that is not compensated; 3) uncontrolled arrhythmias; 4) severe and symptomatic aortic stenosis; 5) hypertrophic cardiomyopathy or cardiomyopathy from recent myocarditis; 6) severe pulmonary hypertension; or 7) other conditions that could be aggravated by exercise (for example, resting systolic blood pressure >200 mm Hg or resting diastolic blood pressure >110 mm Hg; active or suspected myocarditis or pericarditis; suspected or known dissecting aneurysm; thrombophlebitis and recent systemic or pulmonary embolus). In this population no physical activity is recommended for conditioning purposes. Risk stratification for patients with congenital heart disease should be guided by the 26th Bethesda Conference recommendations (28).

TABLE 6   New York Heart Association Classification (8)

Class I   Heart disease without symptoms

Class II   Heart disease with symptoms during ordinary activity

Class III Heart disease with symptoms during less than ordinary activity

Class IV   Heart disease with symptoms at rest

These classifications are presented as a means of beginning exercise with the lowest possible risk. They do not consider accompanying morbidities (for example, insulin-dependent diabetes mellitus, morbid obesity, severe pulmonary disease, complicated pregnancy, or debilitating neurological or orthopedic conditions) that may constitute a contraindication to exercise or necessitate closer supervision during exercise training.

Using Screening Results for Exercise Prescription

For individuals considered to be in Class A, exercise training intensity (Table 4) may be prescribed using the rating of perceived exertion alone and/or specific target heart rates. A suggested rating of perceived exertion for such persons is 12-16 (moderate to hard) on the Borg scale of 6-20 and/or an intensity level that corresponds to 50-90% of maximum heart rate or 45-85% of maximum oxygen uptake or heart rate reserve. Heart rate reserve is defined as maximum heart rate minus resting heart rate. For persons taking medications that affect heart rate (e.g., beta-adrenergic blockers), these heart rate methods do not apply unless guided by an exercise tolerance test.

In the absence of atrial fibrillation, frequent atrial or ventricular ectopy, a fixed-rate pacemaker, or similar conditions, exercise intensity should be prescribed for persons with cardiovascular disease (Class B or C) using target heart rates and perceived exertion ratings in accordance with previously published guidelines (2,8). For these persons, target heart rates should be prescribed using data obtained during exercise testing performed while the participant is taking his or her usual cardioactive medications. In the absence of myocardial ischemia or other significant exercise test abnormalities, a target range of 50-90% of peak heart rate or 45-85% of peak measured oxygen uptake or heart rate reserve is recommended. This intensity level corresponds to 12-16 (moderate to hard) on the Borg scale. In the presence of myocardial ischemia (i.e., ischemic ST-segment depression >1 mm, chest discomfort believed to be angina pectoris, or other symptoms believed to be an anginal equivalent), significant arrhythmia, or other significant exercise test abnormalities (e.g., a fall in systolic blood pressure from baseline, systolic blood pressure >240 mm Hg, or diastolic blood pressure >110 mm Hg), the target training intensity is derived from the heart rate associated with the abnormality. If this occurs at a high level of exercise, the above target heart rate recommendations are applicable, provided that the upper limit of the range is at least 10 beats per minute (bpm) below the level at which the abnormality appears. Otherwise, the recommended upper limit of training heart rate is 10 bpm less than that associated with the abnormality.

STAFFING

Health/fitness facility personnel involved in management or delivery of exercise programs must meet academic and professional standards and have the required experience as established by the ACSM (2,19). Such personnel include the general manager/executive director, medical liaison, fitness director, and exercise leader. In general, health/fitness facility personnel should have the formal training and experience needed to ensure that clients are provided with safe, effective programs and services. The levels of education and experience needed to ensure effectiveness and safety vary with the health status of the client population. The kinds of personnel who should be employed at health/fitness facilities serving various types of clients are summarized in Table 5.

The general manager/executive director is responsible for the overall management of the facility and should have competencies in business as well as design and delivery of exercise programs.

The medical liaison reviews medical emergency plans, witnesses and critiques medical emergency drills, and reviews medical incident reports. In level 2 and 3 facilities (Table 5), the medical liaison may be a licensed physician, a registered nurse trained in advanced cardiac life support, or an emergency medical technician. In level 4 and 5 facilities (Table 5), the medical liaison must be a licensed physician.

The fitness director manages the facility's exercise and activity programs and is responsible for program design and the training and supervision of staff. He or she must have a degree in exercise science, another health-related field, or equivalent experience, and knowledge of exercise physiology, exercise programming, and operation of exercise facilities. The fitness director must hold professional certification at an advanced level by a nationally recognized health/fitness organization. In level 3 facilities this certification should be comparable to ACSM health fitness instructor certification. In level 4 and 5 facilities the fitness director should be certified at a level that correlates with ACSM exercise specialist certification. The exercise specialist typically holds a master's degree in exercise science or a related field and has extensive experience in exercise testing and leadership in clinical populations. He or she must be trained in cardiopulmonary resuscitation (CPR) and should have at least 1 yr of supervisory experience in the fitness industry.

The exercise leader works directly with program participants and provides instruction and leadership in specific modes of exercise. He or she also helps program participants master the behavioral skills needed to adhere to exercise programs. In level 1, 2, and 3 facilities the exercise leader as a minimum must have a high school diploma or equivalent and entry-level or higher professional certification from a nationally recognized health/fitness organization (comparable to ACSM exercise leader certification). In level 4 facilities, the exercise leader should have education and experience corresponding to that required by ACSM health fitness instructor certification. In level 5 facilities, the exercise leader should be either an exercise specialist or a health fitness instructor directly supervised by an exercise specialist. *In all cases the exercise leader must be trained in CPR and should have prior supervised internship or work experience in the health/fitness industry.*

Some health/fitness facilities provide services in allied health fields such as nutrition, stress management, and physical therapy. Personnel providing such services should meet current accepted professional standards in those fields and should be certified as recommended by relevant professional organizations and licensed by or registered with the state as required by law.

EMERGENCY POLICIES AND PROCEDURES

All health/fitness facilities must have written emergency policies and procedures that are reviewed and practiced regularly. Such plans will correspond to the type of facility and risk level of its membership outlined in Table 5. All fitness center staff who directly supervise program participants should be trained in basic life support. Health/fitness facilities must develop appropriate emergency response plans and must train their staff in appropriate procedures to provide during a life-threatening emergency. When an incident occurs, each staff member must perform the necessary emergency support steps in accordance with established procedures. It is important for everyone to know the emergency plan. Emergency drills should be practiced once every 3 months or more often with changes in staff; retraining and rehearsal are especially important. When new staff are hired, new team arrangements may be necessary. Because life-threatening cardiovascular emergencies are rare, constant vigilance by staff and familiarity with the plan and how to follow it are important.

It is essential to acknowledge that emergency equipment alone does not save lives. Equipment alone may offer a false sense of security if it is not backed up with appropriate staffing. The training and preparedness of an astute professional staff who can readily handle emergencies is paramount. This issue is particularly important if persons with certain medical conditions are recruited and encouraged to exercise in a specific health/fitness facility. Such a facility has the responsibility to offer appropriate coverage by personnel as outlined above and in Table 5. Acquisition of equipment for evaluation and resuscitation will depend on the risk level of participants, personnel, and medical coverage. All facilities must have a telephone that is readily accessible and available when emergency assistance is needed. It would be useful for all supervised facilities to have a sphygmomanometer and stethoscope readily available. Level 4 and 5 facilities that recruit members with known cardiovascular disease must have such equipment available, and level 5 (supervised cardiac rehabilitation) facilities should be fully equipped according to the recommendations of the AHA (21) and the American Association of Cardiovascular and Pulmonary Rehabilitation (1). Such equipment includes a defibrillator, oxygen, and fully stocked crash cart. Delineation of specific equipment standards in such facilities is beyond the scope of these guidelines; such information is detailed in the documents above (1,21). Appropriately trained staff who are medically and legally empowered must be available to operate such devices during a facility's operational hours.

The emergency plan must address transportation of victims to a hospital emergency room and must include telephone access to 911 or the local emergency unit access system. Health/fitness facility personnel should be familiar with emergency transport teams in the area so that access and location of the center are clearly identified. Staff should greet the emergency response team at the entrance of the facility so that they can be promptly guided to the site of the emergency. A staff member should remain with the victim at all times. Prompt emergency transport is optimized by free and ready access to the victim within the health/fitness facility and assistance by designated staff.

GENERAL CONSIDERATIONS IN SELECTING A HEALTH/FITNESS FACILITY

In selecting a health/fitness facility, an individual should first consider his or her health status. Persons with a history of cardiovascular disease should seek facilities that provide or require a thorough medical evaluation of prospective members/users. Personnel should include nurses, exercise specialists, health/fitness instructors, and/or exercise leaders licensed or certified by the appropriate agencies, organizations, or authorities. They should be trained to recommend and supervise exercise in patients with cardiovascular and other chronic diseases. Persons at high risk for development of cardiovascular disease should seek facilities that require appropriate medical evaluation of clients and employ exercise leaders who are certified as competent to design and deliver exercise programs for high-risk persons. Table 5 summarizes personnel and safety recommendations for health/fitness facilities (levels 1 through 5) serving clients in various health categories (Classes A through C).

Persons seeking health/fitness facilities should select one that meets professional and industry standards. Facilities should be clean, well-maintained, and spacious enough to ensure the comfort and safety of program participants. Indoor facilities should be climate controlled, and changing rooms and showers should be provided. Flooring in areas where exercise is to be carried out should be designed to minimize risk of injury. Exercise equipment should be well-maintained. The variety, amount, and availability of exercise equipment should match individual needs and preferences, including time of day and preferred mode of exercise. For example, if aerobic dance is the preferred mode of exercise, individuals should seek a fitness center that offers this program at a convenient time and that provides an exercise leader who is competent in this activity and able to teach men and women of various age and fitness levels.

The programs and services of a health/fitness center should optimize participation. The location of the center should minimize time spent traveling to it. The social environment should be attractive and the staff competent in helping members/users master the behavioral skills needed to adopt and maintain a physically active lifestyle.

SUMMARY OF KEY POINTS

- Physical inactivity is a risk factor for cardiovascular disease; it is very prevalent and an important health issue.
- Regular exercise reduces subsequent cardiovascular morbidity and mortality (7,17,18).

- Efforts to promote physical activity will impact everyone, including persons with cardiovascular disease.
- The incidence of a cardiovascular event during exercise among patients with cardiac disease is greater than that among otherwise healthy persons (8).
- Overall, in the general population the absolute incidence of death during exercise is relatively low (8).
- *All facilities offering exercise equipment or services should conduct a cardiovascular screening of all new members and/or prospective users.* Preparticipation screening should identify persons at high risk, and public health efforts should focus on increasing the use of screening. In view of the potential legal risk assumed by operators of fitness facilities, it is recommended that those facilities providing staff supervision document the results of screening.
- When a medical evaluation/recommendation is advised or required, written and active communication by facility staff with the individual's personal physician (or healthcare provider) is strongly recommended.
- Health appraisal questionnaires should be used before exercise testing and/or training to initially classify participants by risk for triage and preliminary decision making. After the initial health appraisal and, if indicated, medical consultation and supervised exercise test, participants can be further classified for exercise training on the basis of individual characteristics.
- Every effort should be made to educate participants about the importance of obtaining a preparticipation health appraisal and, if indicated, a medical evaluation/recommendation. The potential risks incurred without obtaining an appraisal and/or evaluation should also be emphasized.
- *The AHA, the IHRSA, and the ACSM recommend that all health/fitness facilities have written emergency policies and procedures that are reviewed and practiced regularly (16,19).* It is essential to acknowledge that emergency equipment alone does not save lives: training and preparedness by astute professional staff who can readily handle emergencies is paramount.
- Whatever their health status, persons seeking a health/fitness facility should choose one that provides equipment, programs, staff, services,

and membership contracts appropriate for their needs and that meets accepted professional and industry standards.

REFERENCES

1. American Association of Cardiovascular, and Pulmonary Rehabilitation. *Guidelines for Cardiac Rehabilitation Programs*, 2nd Ed. Champaign, IL: Human Kinetics Publishers, 1995.

2. American College of Sports Medicine. *Guidelines for Exercise Testing and Prescription*, 5th Ed., W.L. Kenney (Ed.). Baltimore: Williams & Wilkins, 1995:269-287.

3. American Heart Association. *Heart and Stroke Facts: 1997 Statistical Supplement.* Dallas: AHA, 1996.

4. Anderson, K.M., P.W. Wilson, P.M. Odell, and W.B. Kannel. An updated coronary risk profile: a statement for health professionals. *Circulation* 83:356-362, 1991.

5. Borg, G.A. Psychophysical basis of perceived exertion. *Med. Sci. Sports Exerc.* 14:377-381, 1982.

6. Fletcher, G. How to implement physical activity in primary and secondary prevention: a statement for healthcare professionals from the American Heart Association. *Circulation* 96:355-357, 1997.

7. Fletcher, G.F., G.J. Balady, S.N. Blair, et al. Statement on exercise: benefits and recommendations for physical activity programs for all Americans. *Circulation* 94:857-862, 1996.

8. Fletcher, G.F., G.J. Balady, V.F. Froelicher, L.H. Hartley, W.L. Haskell, and M.L. Pollock. Exercise standards: a statement from the American Heart Association. *Circulation* 91:580-615, 1995.

9. Gibbons, R.J., G.J. Balady, J.W. Beasley, et al. ACC/AHA guidelines for exercise testing: a report of the American College of Cardiology/American Heart Association Task Force on Practice Guidelines. *J. Am. Coll. Cardiol.* 30:260-311, 1997.

10. Healthy People 2000: National Health Promotion and Disease Prevention Objectives. U.S. Dept. of Health and Human Services/Public Health Service. Publication no. (PHS) 91-50213.

11. *How to Choose a Health Club.* Milwaukee, WI: Wisconsin Affiliate, American Heart Association, 1989.

12. Maron, B.J., P.D. Thompson, J.C. Puffer, et al. Cardiovascular preparticipation screening of competitive athletes: a statement for health professionals from the American Heart Association. *Circulation* 94:850-856, 1996.

13. Maron, B.J., J. Shirani, L.C. Poliac, R. Mathenge, W.C. Roberts, and F.O. Mueller. Sudden death in young competitive athletes: clinical, demographic, and pathological profiles. *J.A.M.A.* 276:199-204, 1996.

14. McInnis, K.J., S. Hayakawa, and G.J. Balady. Cardiovascular screening and emergency procedures at health clubs and fitness centers. *Am. J. Cardiol.* 80:380-383, 1997.

15. Mittleman, M.A., M. Maclure, G.H. Tofler, J.B. Sherwood, R.J. Goldberg, and J.E. Muller. Triggering of acute myocardial infarction by heavy physical exertion: protection against triggering by regular exertion. *N. Engl. J. Med.* 329:1677-1683, 1993.

16. *1997 IHRSA/American Sports Data Health Club Trend Report.* Hartsdale, NY: American Sports Data, 1997.

17. Paffenbarger, R.S., R.T. Hyde, A.L. Wing, and C.C. Hsieh. Physical activity, all-cause mortality, and longevity of college alumni. *N. Engl. J. Med.* 314:605-613, 1986.

18. Pate, R.R., M. Pratt, S.N. Blair, et al. Physical activity and public health: a recommendation from the Centers for Disease Control and Prevention and the American College of Sports Medicine. *J.A.M.A.* 273:402-407, 1995.

19. Peterson, J.A., and S.J. Tharrett, eds. *American College of Sports Medicine Health/Fitness Facility Standards and Guidelines,* 2nd Ed. Champaign, IL: Human Kinetics Publishers, 1997.

20. *Physical Activity and Health: A Report of the Surgeon General.* Atlanta: U.S. Department of Health and Human Services, Centers for Disease Control and Prevention, National Center for Chronic Disease Prevention and Health Promotion, 1996.

21. Pina, I.L., G.J. Balady, P. Hanson, A.J. Labovitz, D.W. Madonna, and J. Myers. Guidelines for clinical exercise testing laboratories: a statement for healthcare professionals from the American Heart Association. *Circulation* 91:912-921, 1995.

22. Shephard, R.J., S. Thomas, and I. Weller. The Canadian home fitness test: 1991 update. *Sports Med.* 11:358-366, 1991.

23. Siscovick, D.S., N.S. Weiss, R.H. Fletcher, and T. Lasky. The incidence of primary cardiac

arrest during vigorous exercise. *N. Engl. J. Med.* 311:874-877, 1984.

24. Thomas, S., J. Reading, and R.J. Shephard. Revision of the Physical Activity Readiness Questionnaire (PAR-Q). *Can. J. Sports Sci.* 17:338-345, 1992.

25. Thompson, P.D. The cardiovascular complications of vigorous physical activity. *Arch. Intern. Med.* 156:2297-2302, 1996.

26. Thompson, P.D., E.J. Funk, R.A. Carleton, and W.Q. Sturner. Incidence of death during jogging in Rhode Island from 1975 through 1980. *J.A.M.A.* 247:2535-2538, 1982.

27. Tofler, G.H., J.E. Muller, P.H. Stone, et al. Modifiers of timing and possible triggers of acute myocardial infarction in the Thrombolysis in Myocardial Infarction Phase II (TIMI II) study group. *J. Am. Coll. Cardiol.* 20:1049-1055, 1992.

28. 26th Bethesda Conference. Recommendations for determining eligibility for competition in athletes with cardiovascular abnormalities. *J. Am. Coll. Cardiol.* 24:845-899, 1994.

29. Van Camp, S.P., C.M. Bloor, F.O. Mueller, R.C. Cantu, and H.G. Olson. Nontraumatic sports death in high school and college athletes. *Med. Sci. Sports Exerc.* 27:641-647, 1995.

30. Van Camp, S.P., and R.A. Peterson. Cardiovascular complications of outpatient cardiac rehabilitation programs. *J.A.M.A.* 256:1160-1163, 1986.

31. Willich, S.N., M. Lewis, H. Lowel, H.R. Arntz, F. Schubert, and R. Schroder. Physical exertion as a trigger of acute myocardial infarction. *N. Engl. J. Med.* 329:1684-1690, 1993.

This scientific statement was written by Gary J. Balady M.D., Chair; Bernard Chaitman, M.D., David Driscoll, M.D., Carl Foster, Ph.D., Erika Froelicher, Ph.D., Neil Gordon, M.D., Russell Pate, Ph.D., James Rippe, M.D., and Terry Bazzarre, Ph.D.

ACSM/AHA Joint Position Statement

Automated External Defibrillators in Health/Fitness Facilities

In 1998, the AHA/ACSM published recommendations (5,6) for health/fitness facilities regarding the screening of clients for the presence of cardiovascular disease, appropriate staffing, emergency policies, equipment, and procedures relative to the client base of a given facility. Accordingly, health/fitness facilities are defined as organizations that offer exercise-based health and fitness programs as their primary or secondary service or that promote moderate- to vigorous-intensity recreational physical activity. These range from level 1 (unsupervised exercise room) to level 5 (medically supervised exercise program), and their specific characteristics are outlined in Table 1. Details regarding emergency readiness are provided in the AHA/ACSM recommendations (5,6) and emphasize that all health/fitness facilities must have written emergency policies and procedures that are reviewed and practiced regularly, and that in all supervised facilities, exercise leaders must be trained in basic cardiopulmonary resuscitation (CPR). Because of the publication of the 1998 AHA/ACSM recommendations, 47 states have since passed Good Samaritan legislation, and the federal government has passed the Cardiac Arrest Survival Act and the Rural Access to Emergency Devices Act as components of the federal Public Health Improvement Act of 2000 (7). These state and federal laws now serve to expand Good Samaritan legal protections to users of automated external defibrillators (AEDs) throughout the nation. Therefore, the purpose of this statement is to supplement the 1998 AHA/ACSM recommendations (5,6) regarding the purchase and use of AEDs in health/fitness facilities. Similar to the parent document (5,6), these recommendations are based on a review of the literature and consensus of the writing group after having undergone extensive peer review and final approval by AHA and ACSM. The recommendations are not mandatory or all encompassing, nor do they limit provision of individualized care by health/fitness facilities exercising independent judgment.

This joint position paper was authored by the American College of Sports Medicine and the American Heart Association, and the content appears in AHA style. This paper is being published concurrently in *Medicine & Science in Sports & Exercise* and in *Circulation*. Individual name recognition is reflected in the acknowledgements at the end of the statement.

TABLE 1   Health/Fitness Facilities Emergency Plans and Equipment[a]

	Level 1	Level 2	Level 3	Level 4	Level 5
Type of facility	Unsupervised exercise room (e.g., those in hotels, commercial buildings, and apartment complexes)	Single exercise leader	Fitness center for general membership	Fitness center offering special programs for clinical populations	Medically supervised clinical exercise program (e.g., cardiac rehabilitation)
Personnel[b]	None	• Exercise leader • Recommended: medical liaison	• General manager • Health/fitness instructor • Exercise leader • Recommended: medical liaison	• General manager • Exercise specialist • Health/fitness instructor • Medical liaison	• General manager • Exercise specialist • Health/fitness instructor • Medical liaison
Emergency plan	Present	Present	Present	Present	Present
Emergency equipment	• Telephone in room • Signs • Encouraged: PAD plan with AED as part of the composite PAD plan in the host facility (e.g., hotel, commercial building, apartment complex)	• Telephone • Signs • Encouraged: blood pressure kit, stethoscope, PAD plan with AED	• Telephone • Signs • Encouraged: blood pressure kit, stethoscope, PAD plan with AED (the latter are strongly encouraged in facilities with membership >2,500 and those in which EMS response time is expected to be >5 min from recognition of arrest)	• Telephone • Signs • Blood pressure kit • Stethoscope • Strongly encouraged: PAD plan with AED	• Telephone • Signs • Blood pressure kit • Stethoscope • Oxygen • Crash cart • Defibrillator[c]

AED, automatic external defibrillator; PAD, public access to defibrillator.
[a] This table should replace the bottom half of Table 5 of the AHA/ACSM Recommendations (5,6).
[b] Detailed definitions and competencies for personnel positions are outlined in the ACSM Guidelines (10).
[c] Standard equipment in level 5 facilities includes a defibrillator (5,6,22).

ROLE OF AEDS IN THE CHAIN OF SURVIVAL

An AED is a device that incorporates a rhythm-analysis system and a shock-advisory system for victims of cardiac arrest (1). The AED advises a shock, and the operator must take the final action to deliver the shock. The International Guidelines for Cardiopulmonary Resuscitation and Emergency Cardiovascular Care (2) conclude that early CPR is the best treatment for cardiac arrest until the arrival of an AED and advanced cardiac life support care. The chain of survival includes a series of actions designed to reduce mortality associated with cardiac arrest. Early CPR plays an important role in the chain of survival that includes the following links:

1) early recognition of cardiopulmonary arrest, 2) early CPR, 3) early defibrillation when indicated, and 4) early advanced cardiac life support care (3). Early CPR can prevent ventricular fibrillation from deteriorating to asystole, may increase the chance of successful defibrillation, contributes to the preservation of heart and brain function, and significantly improves survival (4). Importantly, for victims of sudden, shockable cardiac arrest (ventricular fibrillation or pulseless ventricular tachycardia), the single greatest determinant of survival is the time from collapse to defibrillation. A recent review (17) summarizes the data comparing the time-to-shock between first responders (i.e., firefighters, police, and emergency medical system (EMS) basic life support personnel) versus paramedics and dem-

onstrates significantly shorter times among first responders in three of five studies. A survival rate, among victims of witnessed ventricular fibrillation cardiac arrest, as high as 90% has been reported when defibrillation is achieved within the first minute of collapse (8,11,14,15,21). Survival rates decline 7-10% with every minute that defibrillation is delayed, such that a cardiac arrest victim without defibrillation beyond 12 minutes has only a 2-5% chance of survival (1). The highest survival rates for out of hospital cardiac arrest have been reported in cardiac rehabilitation programs equipped with defibrillators (i.e., Table 1: level-5 facilities), where survival approaches 90% (8,11,14,15,21). The International Guidelines (2) conclude that public access to defibrillation (PAD) accomplished by the placement of AEDs in selected locations for immediate use by trained laypersons may be the key intervention to significantly increase survival from an out-of-hospital cardiac arrest. Two recent observational studies report impressive results regarding the effectiveness of PAD in persons with witnessed cardiac arrest, who are in ventricular fibrillation, with AED placement in casinos (20) and on airplanes (19). The cardiac arrest survival rates to discharge from the hospital were 53% and 40%, respectively.

CARDIOVASCULAR RISKS OF EXERCISE

The AHA/ACSM Recommendations (5,6) provide details regarding the cardiovascular risks of exercise. It is clear that the risk of adverse cardiovascular events including death is greater among those individuals with cardiovascular disease than among presumably healthy individuals (5,6,9). As the demographics of the more than 30 million individuals who exercise at health/fitness facilities demonstrate a steady increase in the number of members older than 35 yr (approximately 55% of current membership) (16), it is reasonable to presume that the number of members with cardiovascular disease (and other comorbidities) is rising as well. Although there are no data regarding the incidence of cardiac arrest at health/fitness facilities, two recent surveys provide some important insight. A large database consisting of more than 2.9 million members of a large commercial health/fitness facility chain demonstrates 71 deaths (mean age 52 ± 13 yr; 61 men, 10 women) occurring over a 2-year period, yielding a rate of 1 death/100,000 members/year. The death rate was highest among those members who exercised less frequently, such that nearly half of exercise-related deaths were in those who exercised less than once/week (12). The cardiac arrest rate was not reported but was presumably higher than the death rate. A recent survey of 65 randomly chosen health/fitness facilities in Ohio (18) reports the occurrence of sudden cardiac arrest or heart attack in 17% of facilities during a 5-year period. Notably, only 3% of facilities had an AED on site. Thus, it is prudent to conclude that health/fitness facilities should be considered among the sites in which PAD programs should be established.

RECOMMENDATIONS

It is essential to acknowledge that emergency equipment alone does not save lives. The ACSM/AHA Recommendations (5,6) emphasize the importance of written emergency policies and procedures that are reviewed and practiced regularly. Well-trained health/fitness facility staff members are essential to maintain strong links in the chain of survival for their clients. Effective placement and use of AEDs at all health/fitness facilities (Table 1: levels 1-5) is encouraged, as permitted by law, to achieve the goal of minimizing the time between recognition of cardiac arrest and successful defibrillation. Until further definitive data are available, AED placement is strongly encouraged in those health/fitness facilities with a large number of members (i.e., membership > 2500; [> median size health/fitness facility (16)]); those that offer special programs to clinical populations (i.e., programs for the elderly or those with medical conditions (level 4)) (note that in level-5 facilities, current equipment standards require defibrillators (5,6,22)); and those health/fitness facilities in which the time from the recognition of cardiac arrest until the first shock is delivered by the EMS is anticipated to be > 5 minutes. In unsupervised exercise rooms (level-1 facilities), such as those that might be located in hotels, apartment complexes, or office buildings, the AED should be part of the overall PAD plan for the host facility. At the least, an unsupervised exercise room should have a telephone available in the room with clearly posted numbers to call in case of emergency. In supervised settings, it is essential that designated health/fitness facility staff members who are trained in CPR be present during all hours of operation. CPR should be initiated as soon as a cardiac arrest is recognized and should be continued until the AED is placed on the victim and is activated. In cases of cardiac arrest not due to ventricular fibrillation (VF) or pulseless ventricular tachycardia (VT), AEDs are of no value, and CPR must be maintained. Also, after successful termination of VF/pulseless VT, the rescuer must be able to open the airway and support ventilation and circulation with chest compressions as needed until the arrival of EMS personnel.

Therefore, the establishment of a PAD at all health/fitness facilities is encouraged. This plan should include the following:

- Have written emergency policies and procedures that are practiced regularly (i.e., at least once every 3 months).

- Designate staff members who are trained in CPR and function as first responders in the health/fitness facility setting during all hours of operation.

- Train staff to recognize cardiac arrest.

- Activate EMS—assign staff to meet the emergency response team at the entrance of the facility so that they can be promptly guided to the victim.

- Provide CPR.

- Attach/operate AED (detailed instructions are provided by the specific equipment manufacturer and general recommendations are outlined in the Guidelines 2000 for Cardiopulmonary Resuscitation and Emergency Cardiovascular Care (1)).

- The use of AEDs on infants and children < 8 yr of age is not recommended (1).

Health/fitness facilities should coordinate their PAD program with the local EMS, because many dispatch systems use local phone-directed protocols to assist rescuers in the use of AED and may notify local EMS en route that an AED is being used at the scene. Moreover, the local EMS may assist with program planning and quality improvement, including medical direction, AED deployment and protocols, training, monitoring, and review of AED events (1). Emergency drills should be practiced at least once every 3 months or more often when staff changes occur (5,6). When new staff are hired, new team arrangements may be necessary. The simulated use of AEDs in drills offers the best opportunity for skills maintenance. Maintaining the AED device in proper working condition according to the manufacturer's recommendations is essential. PAD programs must comply with local or regional regulation and legislation.

COSTS

Details regarding the technical aspects of AEDs are available elsewhere (1,17). At present, the cost of an AED is approximately $3000–$4500 per unit. It is expected that the price of AEDs will likely decrease as their use becomes more widespread. The National Heart Lung and Blood Institute (NHLBI), in partnership with the AHA and industry, is conducting a multisite, controlled, prospective study to determine the efficacy and cost-effectiveness of placing AEDs in a variety of public settings. A recent independent study (13) has demonstrated that a program of placing AEDs on large (> 200 passenger) and medium (> 100 passenger) capacity aircraft attain generally accepted levels of cost-effectiveness. However, the cost-effectiveness of AED deployment on smaller aircraft is, at this time, less certain. Similarly, as the cost-effectiveness of AED placement in health/fitness facilities is unknown, it is expected that these recommendations will be reviewed and updated when such data become available. At this time, individual health/fitness facilities are encouraged to maintain data on the utility of their PAD programs and perhaps engage in a collaborative effort with other health/fitness facilities to assess the success of their programs.

SUMMARY OF KEY POINTS

- The Cardiac Arrest Survival Act and the Rural Access to Emergency Devices Act, as components of the federal Public Health Improvement Act of 2000, as well as Good Samaritan laws passed in 47 states, expands Good Samaritan legal protections to users of AEDs throughout the nation.

- The placement of AEDs in selected locations for immediate use by trained laypersons may be the key intervention to significantly increase survival from an out-of-hospital cardiac arrest.

- The chain of survival includes a series of actions designed to reduce mortality associated with cardiac arrest and includes the following links: 1) early recognition of cardiopulmonary arrest, 2) early CPR, 3) early defibrillation when indicated, and 4) early advanced cardiac life support care.

- Well-trained health/fitness facility staff members are essential to maintain strong links in the chain of survival for their clients.

- Effective placement and use of AEDs at all health/fitness facilities (Table 1: levels 1-5) is encouraged, as permitted by law, to achieve the goal of minimizing the time between recognition of cardiac arrest and successful defibrillation. Until further definitive data are available, AED placement is strongly encouraged in those health/fitness facilities with a large number of members (i.e., membership > 2500); those that offer special programs to clinical populations (i.e., programs for the elderly or those with medical conditions (level 4)); and those health/fitness facilities in which the time from the recognition of cardiac arrest until the first shock is delivered by the EMS is anticipated to be > 5 minutes. In unsupervised exercise rooms (level-1 facilities), such as those that might be located in hotels, apartment complexes, or office buildings, the AED should be part of the overall PAD plan for the host facility.

- Health/fitness facilities should coordinate their PAD program with the local EMS.

- Emergency drills should be practiced at least once every 3 months or more often when staff changes occur.

- PAD programs must comply with local or regional regulation and legislation.

This work is a supplement to the AHA/ACSM Recommendations for Cardiovascular Screening, Staffing, and Emergency Policies at Health/Fitness Facilities (5,6).

Writing Group: Gary J. Balady, M.D., Chair; Bernard Chaitman, M.D.; Carl Foster, Ph.D., FACSM; Erika Froelicher, Ph.D.; Neil Gordon, M.D., FACSM; and Steven Van Camp, M.D., FACSM.

REFERENCES

1. American Heart Association and International Liaison Committee on Resuscitation. Guidelines 2000 for Cardiopulmonary Resuscitation and Emergency Cardiovascular Care. *Circulation* 102(Suppl. 1):I60–76, 2000.

2. American Heart Association and International Liaison Committee on Resuscitation. Guidelines 2000 for Cardiopulmonary Resuscitation and Emergency Cardiovascular Care. *Circulation* 102(Suppl. 1):I1–375, 2000.

3. American Heart Association and International Liaison Committee on Resuscitation. Guidelines 2000 for Cardiopulmonary Resuscitation and Emergency Cardiovascular Care. *Circulation* 102(Suppl. 1):I358–370, 2000.

4. American Heart Association and International Liaison Committee on Resuscitation. Guidelines 2000 for Cardiopulmonary Resuscitation and Emergency Cardiovascular Care. *Circulation* 102(Suppl. 1):I22–59, 2000.

5. Balady, G.J., B. Chaitman, D. Driscoll, et al. American Heart Association/American College of Sports Medicine Joint Scientific Statement: Recommendations for Cardiovascular Screening, Staffing, and Emergency Policies at Health/Fitness Facilities. *Circulation* 97:2283–2293, 1998.

6. Balady, G.J., B. Chaitman, D. Driscoll, et al. American Heart Association/American College of Sports Medicine Joint Scientific Statement: Recommendations for Cardiovascular Screening, Staffing, and Emergency Policies at Health/Fitness Facilities. *Med. Sci. Sports Exerc* 30:1009–1018, 1998.

7. Cardiac Arrest Survival Act of 2000. Public Law 106–505, Sec. 401–404.

8. Fletcher, G.F., and J.D. Cantwell. Ventricular fibrillation in a medically supervised cardiac exercise program: clinical, angiographic and surgical correlations. *JAMA* 238:2627–2629, 1977.

9. Fletcher, G.F., G.J. Balady, V.F. Froelicher, L.H. Hartley, W.H. Haskell, and M.L. Pollock. Exercise standards: a statement for health professionals from the American Heart Association. *Circulation* 91:580–615, 1995.

10. Franklin, B. (ed.). *American College of Sports Medicine Guidelines for Exercise Testing and Prescription* (6th Ed.). Baltimore: Williams & Wilkins, 2000, pp. 322–351.

11. Franklin, B.A., K. Bonzheim, S. Gordon, and G.C. Timmis. Safety of medically supervised outpatient cardiac rehabilitation exercise therapy: a 16 year follow-up. *Chest* 114:902–906, 1998.

12. Franklin, B.A., J.M. Conviser, B. Stewart, J. Lasch, and G.C. Timmis. Sporadic exercise: a trigger for acute cardiovascular events? (Abstract). *Circulation* 102(Suppl. 2):II612, 2000.

13. Groeneveld, P.W., J.L. Kwong, Y. Liu, et al. Cost-effectiveness of automated external defibrillators on airlines. *JAMA* 286:1482–1489, 2001.

14. Haskell, W.L. Cardiovascular complications during exercise training of cardiac patients. *Circulation* 57:920–924, 1978.

15. Hossack, K.F., and R. Hartwig. Cardiac arrest associated with supervised cardiac rehabilitation. *J. Cardiac Rehabil.* 2:402–408, 1982.

16. International Health, Racquet, and Sportsclub Association. 2000 Profiles in Success. Boston, 1999.

17. Marenco, J.P., P.J. Wang, M.S. Link, M.K. Homoud, and N.A.M. Estes. Improving survival from sudden cardiac arrest: the role of the automated external defibrillator. *JAMA* 285:1193–1200, 2001.

18. McInnis, K.J., W. Herbert, D. Herbert, J. Herbert, P. Ribisl, and B. Franklin. Low compliance with national standards for cardiovascular emergency preparedness at health clubs. *Chest* 120:283–288, 2000.

19. Page, R.L., J.A. Joglar, R.C. Kowal, et al. Use of automated external defibrillators by a U.S. airline. *N. Engl. J. Med.* 343: 1210–1216, 2000.

20. Valenzuela, T.D., D.J. Roe, G. Nichol, L.L. Clark, D.W. Spaite, and R.G. Hardman. Outcomes of rapid defibrillation by security officers after cardiac arrest in casinos. *N. Engl. J. Med.* 343:1206–1209, 2000.

21. Van Camp, S.P., and R.A. Peterson. Cardiovascular complications of outpatient cardiac rehabilitation programs. *JAMA* 256: 1160–1163, 1986.

22. Williams, M. (ed.). *American Association for Cardiovascular, and Pulmonary Rehabilitation: Guidelines for Cardiac Rehabilitation and Secondary Prevention Programs.* Champaign, IL: Human Kinetics, 1999.

Bibliography

American College of Sports Medicine. *ACSM's guidelines for exercise testing and prescription. 7th Edition.* Philadelphia: Lippincott, Williams and Wilkins; 2006.

American College of Sports Medicine. *ACSM's resource manual for guidelines for exercise testing and prescription. 5th Edition.* Philadelphia: Lippincott, Williams and Wilkins; 2006.

American College of Sports Medicine. *ACSM's health and fitness facility standards and guidelines. 2nd Edition.* Champaign, IL: Human Kinetics; 1997.

American College of Sports Medicine and American Heart Association. *Joint position statement on automated external defibrillators in health/fitness facilities.* 2002.

American Heart Association and American College of Sports Medicine. Joint statement: Recommendations for cardiovascular screening, staffing and emergency policies at health/fitness facilities. *Circulation* 30(6): 1-19. 1998.

American Heart Association. *Guidelines 2000 for cardiopulmonary resuscitation and emergency cardiovascular care. Supplement to Circulation* 102(8); August 2000.

Grantham, W.C.; Patton, R.W.; York, T.D.; Winick, M.L. *Health fitness management.* Champaign, IL: Human Kinetics; 1998.

Herbert, D.L.; Herbert, W.G. *Legal aspects of preventive, rehabilitative and recreational exercise programs. 4th Edition.* Canton, OH: PRC Publishing; 2002.

International Health, Racquet and Sportclub Association. *IHRSA. Global report: State of the health club industry.* Boston: 2002, 2003, 2004, and 2005.

International Health, Racquet and Sportclub Association. *IHRSA's profiles of success.* Boston: 2003 and 2004.

International Health, Racquet and Sportclub Association. *Health and safety, legal and ethical standards for U.S. IHRSA clubs: Standards facilitation guide.* Boston: 1998.

United States Access Board. *Accessible sports facilities: A summary of accessibility guidelines for recreation facilities.* Supplement to Americans with Disabilities Act Access Guidelines. 2002.

United States Access Board. *Accessible swimming pools and spas: A summary of accessibility guidelines for recreation facilities.* Supplement to Americans with Disabilities Act Access Guidelines. 2002.

Tharrett, S. *Fitness management.* Monterey, CA: Healthy Learning; 2005.

INDEX